Praise for The DBT® Solution for Emotional Eating

"The emotional side of out-of-control eating is powerful and real. This easy-to-read, research-based book helps you gain awareness of—and break—the links between emotional distress and food. Highly recommended."
—*Lucene Wisniewski, PhD, private practice, Cleveland, Ohio*

"I'm grateful for this life-changing book. Using the tools in this program, I was able to stop binge eating and also learned emotional awareness skills that have allowed me to make better decisions for myself and my family. I highly recommend it."
—*Linda G., Calgary, Canada*

"This book provides practical strategies and examples, addressing tough issues in a way that puts solutions in anyone's grasp. Very approachable, helpful, and useful."
—*James Lock, MD, PhD, coauthor of* Help Your Teenager Beat an Eating Disorder, Second Edition

"Food meets so many of my emotional needs that the idea of eating less has always been a shock to my system. This book is helping me deal with emotions differently. The tools, details, and practice opportunities I needed are all here."
—*Cori A., San Francisco*

THE DBT® SOLUTION FOR EMOTIONAL EATING

Also Available

Dialectical Behavior Therapy for Binge Eating and Bulimia
Debra L. Safer, Christy F. Telch, and Eunice Y. Chen

The **DBT**® **SOLUTION** for **EMOTIONAL EATING**

A PROVEN PROGRAM TO BREAK THE CYCLE OF BINGEING AND OUT-OF-CONTROL EATING

Debra L. Safer, MD

Sarah Adler, PsyD

Philip C. Masson, PhD

THE GUILFORD PRESS

New York   London

The information in this volume is not intended as a substitute for consultation with healthcare professionals. Each individual's health concerns should be evaluated by a qualified professional.

Printed in the United States of America

This book is printed on acid-free paper.

Last digit is print number: 9   8   7   6   5   4   3   2   1

Library of Congress Cataloging-in-Publication Data is available from the publisher.

ISBN 978-1-4625-2092-3 (paperback) — ISBN 978-1-4625-3302-2 (hardcover)

DBT® is a trademark of Marsha M. Linehan. Marsha M. Linehan has not participated in the preparation of this book.

Contents

Purchasers of this book can download and print enlarged versions of the Diary Card, Behavioral Chain Analysis Form, Steps for Reducing Vulnerability to Emotion Mind worksheet, and Increasing Positive Events worksheet at *www.guilford.com/safer2-forms* for personal use or use with individual clients (see copyright page for details).

Acknowledgments

We are deeply grateful to the many individuals who helped make this book a reality: those serving as therapists and investigators on research trials informing this manual (Therese Elizabeth Kenny, therapist; Christopher W. Singleton, therapist; Kristin von Ranson, PhD, investigator; and Jacquelyn Carter-Major, PhD, investigator), those serving as research assistants (Sarah Pajarito, MS, and Hannah Toyama), and the doctoral students who assisted with the project over the years (including Laurel Wallace, PhD, and Alina Kurland, MS). We also wish to express our sincere appreciation to Craig Forte, LCSW, for his generosity and expertise as a dialectical behavior therapy (DBT) consultant. His intellectual contributions, especially his ability to grasp the more abstract DBT concepts and translate them into everyday language, were invaluable.

We also wish to acknowledge, with deep gratitude, our debt to Marsha M. Linehan, PhD, who inspired us through her own work and specifically encouraged us to test and obtain data regarding this self-help version of our professional manual. Relatedly, we gratefully acknowledge the ongoing influence of the original research by Christy F. Telch, PhD. Her adaptation of DBT for binge eating was the basis for our earlier therapist manual and hence this later self-help version. With pleasure, we also acknowledge our good fortune in having received such skillful guidance from The Guilford Press, especially the dynamic editing duo of Kitty Moore and Christine M. Benton. Their combination of talent, commitment, and unwavering belief in this project's value for patients suffering from emotional eating have been indispensable.

Finally, we want to acknowledge and thank all the individuals who participated in our research trials over the years. This book would not have been possible without you.

*   *   *

I would also like to express my heartfelt appreciation for the love and support of my husband, Adam; daughter, Zoe; parents, Dan and Elaine; parents-in-law, Stanley and Suzanne; and uncle and aunt Howard and Marlene.

DEBRA L. SAFER

I am grateful to my family, who tolerated the many hours I spent away to work on this project, and to all of my many patients, who trusted me to be in their lives.

SARAH ADLER

I acknowledge the unending support of my mother, Patricia; am deeply thankful for the eternal love and encouragement from my partner, Ashley; and will forever appreciate all the teachers, supervisors, and friends whom I have met so far on my journey.

PHILIP C. MASSON

*   *   *

The DBT emotion regulation model of binge eating (pages 18, 21, 24, 25, 33, and 34) is from "Dialectical Behavior Therapy for Depression with Comorbid Personality Disorder" by Thomas R. Lynch and Jennifer S. Cheavens, in *Dialectical Behavior Therapy in Clinical Practice,* edited by Linda A. Dimeff and Kelly Koerner. Copyright © 2007 The Guilford Press. Adapted with permission of The Guilford Press.

The three states of mind (page 73), "Steps for Reducing Vulnerability to Emotion Mind" (page 193), the "Pleasant Events Schedule" (page 197), and "Increasing Positive Events" (page 214) are from *Skills Training Manual for Treating Borderline Personality Disorder* by Marsha M. Linehan. Copyright © 1993 The Guilford Press. Adapted with permission of The Guilford Press.

Introduction

"My eating is out of control."

"I never seem to get full."

"Sometimes I'm in control of my eating, and other times I totally lose it. It's like there's a switch that gets turned on or off."

"When I get overwhelmed, I feel I *have* to eat."

Our relationship with food has a huge impact on the quality of our lives. It can also be quite complicated. In the most straightforward way, food is the fuel our bodies need to keep us alive. But anyone who battles with out-of-control eating knows it isn't quite that simple. Eating is tied to a host of emotions ranging from great pleasure to deep distress. If you have picked up this book, it's very likely that your relationship with food is interfering with the life you want to live and that you're looking for tools to help.

Welcome to the DBT Solution for Emotional Eating

We would like to welcome you to the program. The three of us specialize in treating patients with eating disorders. Debra Safer is a psychiatrist at Stanford University, Sarah Adler is a clinical psychologist also at Stanford University, and Phil Masson is a clinical psychologist with the London Health Sciences Centre in Ontario, Canada. During our training as psychotherapists, each of us was introduced to and particularly impressed with a psychotherapy called dialectical behavior therapy (DBT), which was developed by Marsha Linehan and teaches patients how to manage even their most overwhelming emotions. We have each completed training in DBT and conducted research investigating how the principles of DBT specifically target the emotions that can underlie relationships with food.

This book is a version of DBT that we adapted and tested with patients who were having difficulty controlling their eating. Over the years, we have used this unique approach with over 1,000 patients, and we are excited to be able to offer our collective experience to help you too.

Is This Program a Good Fit for You?

When patients come to our clinic, the first thing we do is ask them to describe what brought them to see us. Over the years patients have described their difficulties with eating using quite a number of different terms, including:

- Binge eating

- Emotional eating

- Compulsive overeating

- Stress eating

- Overeating

- Eating addiction

- Comfort eating

- Out-of-control eating

We don't get too caught up in the specific terms or labels because, when it comes down to it, our patients are struggling and need help. Whether you relate to the terms above or have a different way of thinking about your relationship with food, we ask you to consider how well some of these statements made by our patients may fit you:

- "There's something wrong with me. I'm not like other people—who eat when they're hungry and stop when they're full. I'm never satisfied with normal amounts. I always want more."

- "Food always just seems to call to me. There is no such thing as taking just a taste."

- "Sometimes during a binge I feel like I'm in a trance. Then afterwards I feel awful. I'm embarrassed, demoralized, scared, exhausted, angry, and ashamed—you name it. I vow to myself I will stop and never do it again. I'll even leave tissues on the floor from my tears. But I'll just step over them the next day and do it again. Or maybe I'll stop for a while, but I always end up binge eating again, sooner or later."

- "I hear a lot about being 'addicted' to food. I think there probably are foods I'm addicted to."

- "I'm not sure I even really like food. Food scares me. But I seem to need it to cope with my life. It's not so much it's comforting but it's a distraction that helps me numb out."

- "I'm really frightened about how unhealthy my eating is and how much it's harming my body."

- "I'm afraid that if I continue to misuse food I won't live up to my potential. That I'll never really be happy or at peace with myself."

- "I wonder, can I actually change? I know all of the reasons to change, but I've tried so many times and there is never anything that feels quite as good as food. I don't know if I have the motivation."

If any of these statements sound familiar, this program has been designed for you, as it was for Angela, John, and Leticia.

Angela

"I know I'm an emotional eater. It's rarely about actual physical hunger. Eating comforts me when I'm stressed, calms and distracts me when I'm angry, and is a reward when I'm happy. I feel like I can't resist my urges to overeat no matter how hard I try or how much I tell myself I'll regret it. And most of the time my overeating turns into a binge and I feel physically sick. I can't tell you how many times I've promised I'll stop, but then I do it again. Other people seem to be able to handle things I can't without eating. Why can't I? I feel trapped and stuck!"

John

"I simply lack self-control. I have no idea what sets me off. I can just be hanging out at home watching TV and suddenly I'm finishing off more than a pint of ice cream. Nothing is going on at the time, it just seems like binge eating is a bad habit, something I fall into when I'm bored and want to relax, wind down. I don't know what's wrong with me. I can get myself to change other bad habits, but this one feels impossible."

Leticia

"I've been struggling with my weight my entire life. I love to eat, and I seem to have no control, especially over certain foods. Carbs are my enemy!

Even when I make a decision I won't overeat, I'll eat one thing that's off my plan and just end up giving up and totally blowing it. Like, the minute the bread basket comes to the table I'll have one slice, and then it seems I can't stop. Or, whatever it is, I can't seem to have any control once I'm off track. It's always black and white—I'm on my diet or I'm off. I can't stand how much this struggle has dominated my life. I don't know how to just eat normally."

If you identify with Angela's, John's, or Leticia's story, this program could be an excellent fit for you. You'll get a lot of help from their experiences, which we will follow throughout this book to show how they used this program to dramatically change their eating behaviors and hence the quality of their lives. Their stories are composites representing common experiences of patients we have worked with and are thoroughly disguised to protect their privacy. You'll also be reading the responses to exercises and homework from a patient we call Kat, who graciously gave us permission to use her words (although any identifying details, including her name, have been changed).

Why DBT?

DBT is an extensively researched, effective treatment that teaches practical yet powerful skills to help individuals with difficulty tolerating emotions.

Over the years our patients have told us that they often binge eat, which is commonly defined as eating with a lack of control, in response to discomfort. They've told us they've binged after a disagreement with a loved one, after a very stressful day at work, while staying at home feeling lonely and bored, after trying on clothing that didn't fit, when they were sick or in pain, and even after a date that went really well (feeling excited can feel uncomfortable!). Whatever the specific situation they've described to us, the common element is how the events led to physiological sensations that felt difficult to tolerate or even felt unbearable. Some of our patients readily described these sensations as emotions—such as hurt, anger, happiness, shame, hopelessness, anxiety, and/or desire. Other patients were less aware of what they were feeling, perhaps only able to recall a sense of restlessness or discomfort. Others have started our program without any sense of their emotions at all. According to the DBT model used in this program, binge eating functions by alleviating the discomfort or offering a way to temporarily diminish or avoid uncomfortable sensations. In the long run, however, turning to food as an escape leads to deep regret, sadness, and shame, which decreases self-confidence and can increase the likelihood that our patients turn to food again the next time they are distressed.

Does this sound familiar?

This DBT self-help program for binge eating focuses on the relationship between your feelings and your urges to use food in ways you regret or that are interfering with your life. You will learn three modules, or categories, of DBT skills: **mindfulness, emotion regulation,** and **distress tolerance.** The skills in these modules build on each other. **Mindfulness** skills will help you increase your awareness and stay attuned to why you eat so that, when you're stressed, you can choose behaviors that serve you better than turning to food. **Emotion regulation** involves not only accepting but also learning to influence your emotions by becoming less vulnerable to uncomfortable emotions. **Distress tolerance** will teach you skills for dealing with discomfort in new ways that give you time to reflect and make better choices.

After you complete this program, you will have many, many other skills for coping with your emotions. This will change your relationship with food and help you live a healthier, happier life.

As we mentioned above, DBT has a wealth of research data supporting its effectiveness for many different disorders and problem behaviors, but our studies have focused on showing its effectiveness specifically for patients with disordered eating (details on the research are in the appendix). One of our earliest efforts translated what we learned into a therapists' manual (with coauthors Christy Telch and Eunice Chen) to ensure that the treatment from our research studies would be available to other therapists and clinical investigators.

Then, to make this program more widely available, we wrote a self-help version so that people could learn the skills by working through this book on their own (pure self-help) or with the help of a therapist (guided self-help). Because many self-help manuals that are based on therapist-delivered interventions have not been tested, we designed a study using this book with 60 patients, guided by a therapist, and found it gratifyingly effective:

- After 13 weeks, 40% of those who received the program (and 50% of those who completed it) had fully stopped binge eating compared to only 3% of those who were waiting to start the program.

- Six months later, almost 70% of the original participants who had stopped binge eating by 13 weeks remained binge free.

- Even those patients who did not completely stop binge eating had significant decreases in their binge eating.

So, are we saying that our program, through the use of this book, is your only hope for addressing binge-eating–type problems? Definitely not (see the box on page 7).

What If You Don't Really Identify with the Term *Binge Eating* and Don't Think You Use Food to Soothe Your Emotions?

To date, the best evidence for this program is its effectiveness for patients who have been diagnosed with binge-eating disorder and also for patients with bulimia nervosa who are being treated by a therapist. We are currently carrying out additional research using this program in both self-help and guided self-help formats.

According to the American Psychiatric Association's *Diagnostic and Statistical Manual* (fifth edition, 2013), an episode of binge eating essentially involves feeling out of control while eating a lot more food than most people would within that time period. For binge-eating disorder to be diagnosed, the episodes have to have gone on for a few months. Likewise, bulimia involves out-of-control eating over a period of months, combined with behaviors like vomiting or using laxatives intended to head off the resulting weight gain. But as we said before, we're not overly concerned with labels, and if you've never been diagnosed with one of these disorders and think of your problem in a different way, you can still benefit from this program. The term "binge eating" just doesn't resonate with everyone. Sometimes people call their problems with food "emotional eating." Others describe a pattern in which they tend to "graze" continuously on small amounts of food, despite not feeling hungry. Yet other patients feel they eat without paying attention to what they are eating. They call themselves "mindless eaters" and feel their mindless eating serves an emotional function. We've also worked with many patients who've had weight-loss surgery. Although typically they are physically incapable of eating large amounts of food in single episodes, they ask for help with impulsive choices such as unplanned snacks, overly large mealtime portions, and eating foods not included on the plans provided by their dieticians.

What we really care about is that you are not happy about your relationship with food and that learning skills to help you regulate your urges will help.

It is also our clinical experience that the skills in this program help those with problem behaviors like overspending, overexercising, and overworking (being a "workaholic") that are triggered by emotional distress. You'll meet people struggling with these problems later in the book.

As you can probably see, the consistent thread in this discussion of eating disorders is the link between distressing emotions and binge eating. But what if you're not aware of trying to manage emotional distress by eating in a way you end up regretting? Some of our patients are not aware of what they were feeling before they start to eat. Maybe they came from a family where expressing emotions wasn't acceptable, or even safe, so they avoid knowing how they feel. Often it's not that these patients don't experience strong emotions, but that when they start to feel, they quickly do something to reduce those feelings. This could involve

Other Options: CBT and IPT

We strongly believe that access to tested treatments is important, but unfortunately not all approaches used by clinicians have been shown to be effective for binge eating and bulimia. That's one of the reasons we wanted to make this program, which we researched, available in a guided self-help format. You can find out which treatments for eating disorders have empirical support (found effective in research studies) by visiting MedlinePlus (National Library of Medicine: *http://medlineplus.gov*; in Spanish: *http://medlineplus.gov/spanish*). At the time of this writing, these two have the most empirical support:

• **Cognitive-behavioral therapy (CBT):** The best studied of the empirically supported treatments, CBT conceptualizes strict dieting or other rigid rules about what food is eaten and when as key to the development and maintenance of binge eating. CBT treatment, which has been researched with therapist-led as well as both guided and self-help formats (see Christopher Fairburn's excellent *Overcoming Binge Eating*), involves filling out daily food logs to track the relationship between restrictive eating and binge episodes. While it's quite successful for many individuals, some patients continue to have disordered eating symptoms at the end of CBT treatment. (This is one of the reasons we developed our DBT program, which focuses squarely on the link between difficulty managing emotions and turning to binge eating to temporarily relieve emotional distress. Some of our patients tell us that they don't engage in strict dieting and that most of their binge eating seems to take place despite having eaten regular meals and at times when they aren't physically hungry.)

• **Interpersonal psychotherapy (IPT):** Another well-studied empirically supported treatment, IPT focuses on the connection between interpersonal difficulties and the development and maintenance of binge eating. To date, IPT is not available in a self-help format.

grabbing a snack or turning on the television or checking Facebook. Starting this program and finishing even the first portion of this book has helped these people learn to be more aware of their emotions. As they learn to accept their feelings, without judgment, they identify the link between their feelings and their urges to eat. When they identify the link, they have a much better chance of breaking it.

We are not, of course, implying that this book can help with every type of problem related to emotions or disordered eating. We would definitely not recommend this book as a stand-alone treatment for anorexia nervosa (characterized by low body weight due to ongoing restriction of caloric intake). If you have been diagnosed with anorexia nervosa or are concerned that you may have symptoms, **consult a therapist and physician to come up with a treatment plan designed for your condition, as we are not aware of evidence that self-help approaches are effective.**

What Exactly Does DBT Offer That Other Approaches Don't?

Other approaches that help with binge eating may include attention to emotions, but DBT is the only program that focuses so primarily on the link between emotion dysregulation and binge eating. Central to DBT is that individuals turn to food to self-soothe, numb, and avoid emotional discomfort because food "works" temporarily despite its longer-term negative consequences. As mentioned above, one of the most potent aspects of DBT is that it will teach you specific *skills and strategies* to help you cope with difficult emotions without turning to food. Additionally, DBT incorporates *dialectical thinking*. Dialectical thinking is a flexible mindset that enables you to hold contradictory viewpoints simultaneously, such as recognizing the need to stop binge eating while accepting yourself as you are in this moment. You will also learn a step-by-step method for completing a *behavioral chain analysis*, an amazingly effective way of examining what keeps you stuck in destructive eating patterns. Essentially, we teach you how to become your own DBT coach, fully equipped by the end of the program to practice and maintain the skillful behaviors you need for a healthy relationship with food.

How Should You Use This Book?

Some books are great for flipping through and finding parts that are relevant for you. This is *not* one of those books. We recommend you use this program by reading it in order and working through each chapter. As we mentioned earlier, the skills we will teach you build on each other. Also, each chapter will teach you new skills, and the more skills you have, the more confident you will feel about controlling binges and other problem behaviors, including those that may not involve food. In short, by working through the complete program, you'll have a strong arsenal to help you develop a healthier and happier relationship with food. To give you a sense of how much you'll be learning, we've put together a preview of what each chapter will teach you ("What You Will Learn in This Program: Preview of Upcoming Chapters," pages 11–15).

Each chapter contains exercises and "homework" assignments to guide you in practicing and thinking about the material you're learning. It typically takes most people about a week or two to read a chapter, complete the exercises within, and do the homework at the end of the chapter. If it takes you longer to complete some chapters, that's fine. The vital part of this program is completing each chapter's exercises and homework. In general, though, one chapter every week or two (including homework) is a good rule of thumb.

As you work your way through the book, you'll keep practicing skills you learned in previous chapters. We will be asking you to check off boxes at the end of each chapter indicating that you've practiced the new skills you're accumulating. This way you'll keep reinforcing your old skills while learning new skills to stop your binge eating.

It's also helpful to write directly in this book, and we've allowed space for you to do so throughout. This will make it easier to review, especially in Chapters 7 and 13, in which we help you assess the progress you have made about halfway through and at the end of this program. (If you need more space, feel free to continue recording your thoughts on a separate sheet of paper and tuck it into the book in the appropriate place.)

We have seen firsthand that the patients who read the material and tackle the exercises (don't just read them) get the very most from this program. It *is* an investment, but over time the skills you learn start to become second nature. And the quality of life you create when you are no longer dominated by your relationship with food is priceless!

If you make the commitment to work through this book diligently, investing time every day, the program can be effective as pure self-help. But for some, working with a therapist can increase accountability and lead to greater success. If you decide to use a guided self-help approach, read through the box on page 10. We suggest sharing it with your therapist.

If you don't have or want a therapist but know that you are the kind of person who does better with social support, you might consider asking a trusted person or persons to support you while working through this program.

Will This Program Focus on Weight Loss?

Many patients who binge eat also want to lose weight. This is understandable given both the health consequences and society's negative attitudes toward overweight and obesity. We have found the majority of binge eaters to be dissatisfied with their bodies regardless of size, which can make what we are about to say especially difficult to hear. Our years of experience support the overwhelming research to focus first on stopping your binge eating before considering weight loss. If you've struggled with your weight, you know that losing and keeping weight off is one of the hardest things to do. Dieting inherently involves restriction, and we see that when our patients try to restrict their eating it often sets them up to binge more. Maybe you have observed this if you have tried to diet. We also have observed that when our patients are attempting to follow a rigid diet, they simply can't take advantage of the opportunity to learn and apply the skills we teach. Even when they are able to successfully lose weight, their chance of regain will be even higher because they have not learned to stop binge eating. For these reasons and others, we highly recommend stopping binge eating as the best strategy for long-term weight control. This program, therefore, does not include a focus on weight loss. We discuss this in more detail in Chapter 10 in a section that addresses balanced eating (pages 176–178). If you are currently attempting to follow a restrictive food plan to lose or keep off weight, or are thinking about doing so, we suggest you read this section now before moving ahead.

We look forward to guiding you through this program to help you stop binge eating and transform your life. So, let's get going!

Setting Up Your Own Guided Self-Help Program

So far, research has not told us exactly which elements make guided self-help effective. It's not clear, for example, if the therapist needs to be trained in the treatment. From what we know from the available research, we suggest that you do the following when you look for a therapist (or other trusted, supportive person) to work with you:

1. Tell the therapist your plan to work through this program while meeting with him or her at least every 2–3 weeks.

2. Ask for support in the following areas:

   • Setting a schedule for reading through the self-help program and sticking to the schedule.

   • Identifying any obstacles that are getting in the way of your use of the program and problem solving a plan to address these. For example, a typical obstacle we help our patients with is not using the skills and strategies when they need them.

   • Talking through how to apply the skills to your specific situation, such as by reviewing a behavioral chain analysis.

   • Talking through parts of the program if you don't understand them.

If the therapist agrees to focus on these areas and you feel you have a good working relationship, you will be in a good position to work on this program with support. Having a therapist or other trusted person to help you be accountable can be very helpful.

What You Will Learn in This Program

PREVIEW OF UPCOMING CHAPTERS

In Chapter 1, "The DBT Approach to Stopping Binge Eating," you'll learn:

- How emotions and binge eating are linked and why stopping binge eating is so challenging (the DBT emotion regulation model)

- How biological and environmental factors interact to make some individuals but not others vulnerable to binge eating (the DBT biosocial theory)

- How this program teaches you new skills to use as an alternative to binge eating when you experience difficult emotions

In Chapter 2, "Making a Commitment to Stop Binge Eating," you'll learn:

- How to learn from your past successes and challenges about what works for you and what does not

- To compare the pros and cons of binge eating and imagine what your life would look like if you stopped

- A method for exploring the values you hold most dear and whether binge eating is in line with the life you want for yourself

- The power of making a commitment to stop both binge eating and related problem behaviors

- To understand the importance of making a commitment to this program

- To make a commitment to yourself to stop binge eating (don't worry, we'll discuss this a lot first!)

**In Chapter 3, "Discussing Program Goals and the Tools to Get You There,"
you'll learn:**

- The program's goals and steps

- How to use the Diary Card to keep track of your progress

- The skill of renewing your commitment (pros/cons), the first skill on the
  Diary Card

- How mindfulness skills can help you become less emotionally reactive

- How you can become your own wise mind by balancing your emotional
  and rational responses and make decisions in line with your values

- Diaphragmatic breathing, a simple yet powerful skill that disrupts physical
  reactions that often accompany strong emotions to help you stop binge
  eating

In Chapter 4, "Learning to Become Your Own DBT Coach," you'll learn:

- How to become your own DBT coach by analyzing your binge eating with
  the behavioral chain analysis

- What the behavioral chain analysis is and why it is so important

- How to use the behavioral chain analysis to identify ways to increase your
  chances of stopping a binge

**In Chapter 5, "The Benefits of Dialectical Thinking and Mindfulness," you'll
learn:**

- The benefits of dialectical thinking as an alternative to rigid thinking

- How to apply dialectical thinking to your commitment to stop binge eating
  and use it to help you accept yourself, and to help you tolerate ambivalent
  feelings about stopping binge eating

- The mindfulness skill of observing, which involves beginning to "just
  notice" your experience without getting caught up in it, judging it, or
  reacting to it

- How to use observing to get in touch with your wise mind by paying attention to both physical sensations and emotions

- How to use the skills of dialectical thinking and observing to stop yourself
  from binge eating

In Chapter 6, "Becoming a More Skillful Observer," you'll learn:

- The mindfulness skill of adopting a nonjudgmental stance, or observing your experiences without labeling them or yourself in moral terms such as good or bad, and right or wrong

- The mindfulness skill of focusing on one thing in the moment, or bringing your full awareness and attention to the present, or current moment

- The mindfulness skill of being effective, or focusing on doing what works in order to achieve your goals, instead of getting overly caught up in "being right" or "being perfect"

- How these skills, in conjunction with observing, can help you access your wise mind and stop binge eating

In Chapter 7, "Staying on Track," you'll learn:

- How to practice adopting a nonjudgmental stance while reviewing your progress halfway through the program

- How to use recommendations to make the program even more effective for you

- Which skills have been most useful and which you should use more often

- To review the behavioral chain analysis tool and reflect on what else you can do to stop any remaining binge eating

In Chapter 8, "Mindful Eating and Urge Surfing," you'll learn:

- Mindful eating, the skill of being fully aware and in the moment while you are eating

- Urge surfing, a skill to help you break the connection between having an *urge* to binge eat and *actually* binge eating

In Chapter 9, "Being Mindful of Your Current Emotion and Radically Accepting Your Emotions," you'll learn:

- About emotion regulation skills, a new module that builds on your mindfulness skills but adds new skills that allow you to more directly influence your emotional experience

- Two emotion regulation skills: mindfulness of your current emotion and radically accepting your emotions

- Mindfulness of your current emotion involves using mindfulness skills such as focusing on one thing in the moment to help you decrease the intensity of painful emotions

- Radically accepting your emotions involves a deep and fundamental acceptance of your emotions, including those that are painful, uncomfortable, and/or unpleasant

In Chapter 10, "Reducing Vulnerability to Emotion Mind and Building Mastery," you'll learn:

- How reducing your vulnerability to emotion mind can help you be less vulnerable to binge eating

- How remembering the acronym PLEASE can help you reduce your vulnerability to your emotion mind. These methods include remembering to:

  - Treat *PhysicaL illness*

  - Balance your *Eating*

  - *Avoid* mood-altering substances

  - Balance your *Sleep*

  - Get *Exercise*

- How the skill of building mastery, or engaging in activities that increase your confidence and competence, also reduces your vulnerability to emotion mind

In Chapter 11, "Building Positive Experiences: Steps for Increasing Positive Emotions," you'll learn:

- The importance of actively creating more positive than negative or neutral experiences in your life

- Various ways to increase positive experiences, such as increasing daily pleasant activities, building long-term positive goals, attending to your relationships, and stopping patterns of avoidance ("avoiding avoiding")

- How to increase your enjoyment of the positive experiences you do have by increasing your mindfulness of positive emotions

In Chapter 12, "Distress Tolerance," you'll learn:

- Distress tolerance, a set of skills designed to help you cope during situations of high stress and emotion; the goal is to deal with these stresses without making things worse, such as by binge eating

- More about radical acceptance, a skill involving choosing to accept both yourself and the current situation as it is, without necessarily approving of it

- Half-smiling, a powerful skill that facilitates inner acceptance through relaxing your outer facial muscles

- Three crisis survival skills to help get you through crises, both big and small: distraction (temporarily refocusing outside of yourself to get a needed break, e.g., with activities), self-soothing (finding ways to comfort yourself through your five senses, such as listening to beautiful music), and thinking of pros and cons (giving yourself a chance to think through the pros and cons of tolerating a distressing situation using effective coping skills instead of binge eating)

In Chapter 13, "Reviewing, Planning for the Future, and Preventing Relapse," you'll:

- Review this program's approach and the skills taught, with a focus on those skills you found most helpful

- Review your progress in reducing your binge eating

- Learn a new skill, coping ahead, to prevent binge eating and relapse

- Identify and address any barriers to continuing to build the life you want

1

The DBT Approach to Stopping Binge Eating

Over our many years working with patients we have found that stopping out-of-control eating is one of the hardest things most people will ever do. But don't worry: This program is all about teaching you that *hard* is not the same as *impossible*. It includes three important components:

1. The program starts by explaining why it's such a challenge to stop binge eating. Understanding what triggers a binge and what keeps you trapped in the binge-eating cycle can free you from judging yourself negatively, which actually thwarts your efforts to stop bingeing.

2. Then you'll learn skills and strategies for managing emotions without turning to food. By the end of this program you'll have a whole toolbox of skills to help you face problems instead of avoiding them, tackle them effectively instead of using the destructive approach of binge eating, and manage emotional distress when you encounter one of life's unsolvable problems. Our patients often tell us they think of the program's skills as a kind of "Emotions 101," or a basic life skills course they never had before.

3. The program uses *dialectical thinking*, which provides an alternative to rigid or "black-and-white" patterns that can keep you stuck. Dialectical thinking promotes more flexible thinking and allows you to embrace seemingly contradictory actions that help move you forward—accepting yourself as you are while simultaneously attempting to change, and using skills you already have while remaining open to learning the new ones taught in this program.

The DBT Emotion Regulation Model: Understanding the Link between Emotions and Binge Eating

You may or may not already be aware that you turn to extra food in response to emotional discomfort. The DBT emotion regulation model of binge eating (at the bottom of this page) helps explain how this response unfolds. Emotion *regulation* involves knowing what you're feeling and modulating your reaction to your emotional state or accepting and tolerating it when your emotions can't be changed immediately. According to the model, instead of regulating your emotions you turn to binge eating when your emotions feel too intense to modulate, tolerate, or otherwise manage—when you're emotionally *dysregulated*. Whether your emotions are "positive" (like happiness, excitement, desire), "negative" (like fury, disappointment, worry), or a combination, binge eating has become a learned behavior that serves the function of reducing your emotional distress. The good news is that a learned behavior can be *un*learned. (See the box on the facing page.)

Angela's Story

Angela was driving home late from work thinking about how her boss had criticized her report, leaving her hurt and angry. Brooding over how she

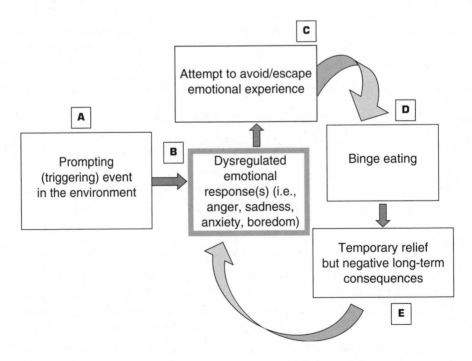

The DBT emotion regulation model of binge eating.

"The Carrot and the Stick": The Fundamentals of Positive and Negative Reinforcement Science

Behavioral psychology helps to explain how reinforcement affects our actions. A reinforcer is anything that increases the chance that we will engage in a behavior. Reinforcers can be positive or negative. A *positive reinforcer* might be being paid money at the end of each binge-eating episode, where a negative reinforcer might be reducing your emotional discomfort. Either reward will encourage you to binge eat again. But, many of our patients argue, they actually feel worse after a binge and it doesn't always "work" to reduce negative, painful emotions. How, then, can reinforcement principles explain why they still binge?

There are two reasons:

1. Bingeing offers the short-term benefit of numbing painful emotions, even though in the longer term it may increase distress, guilt, shame, and disgust.

2. Bingeing seems to "work" some of the time. If it worked every time and then suddenly stopped working, you would probably try something else to deal with painful emotions. But when it "pays off" just often enough to convince you that there's a chance it will do so this time, you'll keep turning to it. Fortunately, you can use this intermittent or variable reinforcement to make positive changes in this program: If you try hard to use the skills we teach in this program and find that sometimes they work very well, you'll be more likely to keep using them even if they don't work every single time.

hadn't gotten clear instructions or the appropriate appreciation for getting so much done alone, in so little time, she felt more and more resentful. As she spotted a fast-food restaurant, she found herself ordering two cheeseburgers, a milk shake, a large fries, and two apple pies. While eating, she stopped thinking about work or how angry she felt. Not too long after, however, she was flooded with disgust and shame. "How come I keep doing this to myself? Why can't I handle anything?" As the night went on she felt more and more furious with herself and increasingly devastated, hopeless, and angry, especially when she thought about having to go back to work the next day. Then she glimpsed her daughter's leftover birthday cake in the fridge and couldn't resist. "It's all too much," she said to herself. She finished the cake, feeling even more ashamed and an even deeper sense of despair. She went to sleep telling herself, "I HAVE to stop. This is crazy. What is wrong with me?"

Despite Angela's determination to stop binge eating, at her core she feels powerless to change because she doesn't truly understand why she's bingeing. We've filled in the DBT emotion regulation model for her first binge on the top of the facing page and for her second binge at the bottom to show not only what led to these binges but also what keeps her caught in this binge-eating cycle.

A: As shown for Angela's first binge, first *something happens.* At this point, Angela's binge eating may seem so automatic that she's not aware of anything setting it off—she just finds herself in the drive-through. But actually, there was a prompting (*triggering*) event (A), which can then lead to certain thoughts and feelings. Here the prompting event was criticism from Angela's boss, which led to the thought "My boss doesn't appreciate me. I'm never treated fairly" and the emotion of anger.

B: This next step is critical. The prompting or triggering event sets off an *emotion* (B) with which you don't feel able to cope. For Angela, it was feeling angrier and angrier at her boss's treatment of her. What types of emotions tend to be hard for you to cope with? Being bored when you are in the house alone might make you feel quite uncomfortable in and of itself. Also, being alone could set off more powerful emotions such as intense sadness, deprivation, or frustration. Even positive emotions like joy or desire can feel uncomfortable if you don't know how to manage their intensity. The idea here is that Angela has begun to experience an emotion that brings her discomfort.

Triggering events can be hard to identify, but essentially they are environmental prompts that start a chain reaction leading to binge eating. Here are a few examples:

> *Prompt:* Catching a glimpse of your reflection. *Thought:* "I look so fat." *Emotion:* Shame.
> *Prompt:* Your spouse flirting with an attractive stranger at a party. *Thought:* "He never looks at me that way anymore." *Emotions:* Sadness, jealousy.
> *Prompt:* Cupcakes from your favorite bakery brought to the office for a birthday. *Thought:* "That would taste SO good! It's not fair that I have to limit how much I eat!" *Emotions:* Resentment, sadness.
> *Prompt:* Eating something off your food plan. *Thought:* "I've already blown it. I might as well keep going." *Emotions:* Resignation or hopelessness.

You may not recognize any of these as triggers when they arise. Even seemingly irrelevant events can become triggers when you're already vulnerable due to sleep deprivation, chronic stress, depression, and so forth.

C: Because intense emotions can be very difficult to deal with, it makes sense that Angela would try to reduce, avoid, or get rid of hers (C). People use a wide

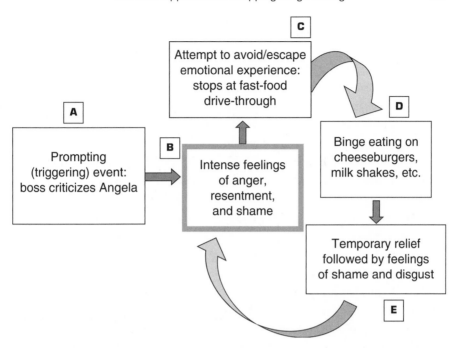

Angela's DBT emotion regulation model for her first binge.

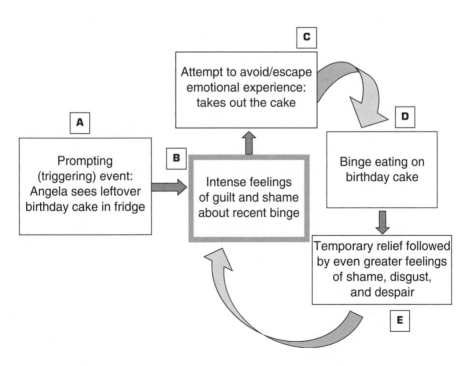

Angela's DBT emotion regulation model for her second binge.

range of strategies to try to feel better, but Angela never learned the skills needed to monitor, evaluate, change, and accept intense emotional experiences.

D: This is why Angela decides to stop off at the fast-food drive-through. Food *temporarily* "solves" her problem, helping her numb out and forget about how angry her boss made her feel. Turning to food reduces her anger, sadness, frustration, loneliness, and any other uncomfortable feelings she has about her boss's actions.

E: But by the time she gets home, Angela begins to feel disgusted with herself and ashamed of her binge eating (E). When the emotions she escaped by binge eating start to creep back in along with the disgust and shame for turning to food, Angela feels even worse.

A: This is when she sees her daughter's birthday cake, which becomes the next prompting event (A) that perpetuates the cycle and sets off her second binge.

B: The uncomfortable emotions are the intense guilt and shame she feels about having turned to food.

C: To avoid or escape from the emotional discomfort, she is overcome with strong urges to take out the birthday cake.

D: She has her second binge, this time on the leftover cake.

E: Though temporarily numbed after eating the cake, by the end of the evening she is even more disgusted with herself and has an even deeper sense of hopelessness and despair.

She tries to feel better by promising herself she "will never do this again." Unfortunately, this promise increases her vulnerability to her intense emotions because she is now depriving herself of the one strategy she had to feel better— eating. She has, in fact, set herself up to repeat the cycle.

Angela experienced an array of intense and uncomfortable emotions. She may, as many people do, believe that her *feelings* are the problem—they are too much, too intense, there is something wrong with her. (As it turns out, people with binge-eating problems may very well be born experiencing emotions more intensely than others, and they may also believe it is inappropriate to experience certain emotions, such as anger. We will discuss this more a little later in this chapter.) However, we believe it's not Angela's feelings that are the problem. Angela's uncomfortable emotions make sense given the situation. When treated unfairly, she feels bad. We believe the problem is the behavior or strategy (binge eating) she is using to cope with her emotions. In the short run, it helps her feel better, but in the long run, her behaviors around food seriously impair her quality of life, leading to more distress, more misery, and more out-of-control eating. Because she doesn't think she has the tools she needs to identify and solve her underlying problem, she gets caught in a vicious cycle that involves not only increasing reliance on binge eating to temporarily manage emotional discomfort but also isolation and a reduced chance of receiving validation, help, and support.

Numbing emotions with food interferes with developing healthy behaviors that may lead to true improvements in your life.

What if you aren't sure whether your emotions are driving your overeating? Maybe you think to yourself, "I just really love eating" or "I just eat when I'm bored." Or maybe you don't know why you overeat. Let's look at John's experience.

John's Story

John is a busy executive with multiple business dinners a week. When he gets home, he sits down on the sofa and turns on the TV. He doesn't feel hungry ("I just ate a big dinner"), but the next thing he knows he is grabbing a pint of ice cream and a spoon. He came to us for help with what he views as an irrational, distressing habit. "Why are you eating?" he demanded of himself. "There's no reason to eat this much. How can you be able to control other things but be such a failure at controlling your eating?"

The DBT emotion regulation model helped John see that binge eating might be more than just an "irrational habit" for him. Recalling that his father had responded to any expression of negative or painful emotions with angry demands to "Stop complaining!" John joked that the only time you were "allowed to complain was if you were so ill you needed to go to the hospital." Because he was motivated to gain control over his binge eating, John was open to the idea that his emotions might be linked to his binge eating. He started paying more attention to what was going on inside of him when he binged. After his most recent binge on ice cream after a business dinner, he was able to break down his "irrational habit" as follows (see page 24).

A: Prompting event: sitting on the sofa with the remote control.

B: There he noticed that his body and mind felt restless—"not wanting to go to bed but not quite knowing what to do with my energy." Internally, he was saying to himself: "I need something, I need something, I need something." As we encouraged him to try to come up with emotion words, he said: "Frustrated. I'm annoyed and frustrated. I spend every waking hour at work or at these work dinners. I come home and go to sleep, and then I start all over again." We asked John if perhaps when he said he "needed something" he could be feeling that work alone wasn't enough. He said that might be true, but it was hard for him to know for sure.

C: John goes to the freezer and takes out the ice cream. His first swallows of ice cream taste delicious, distracting him from his distress. This leads him to continue to eat, although he tells himself harshly to stop.

D: Ultimately, he ends up binge eating the ice cream. In the short run, the

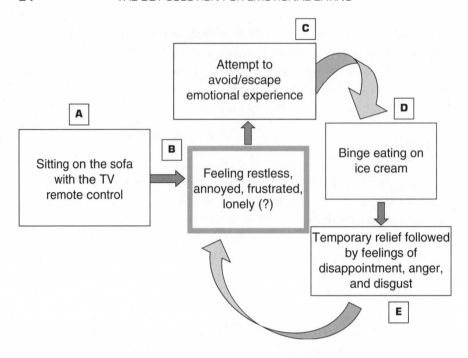

John's DBT emotion regulation model for a binge.

binge allows him to numb himself from the discomfort of restlessness, annoyance, frustration, and other emotions, potentially including feeling empty or lonely.

E: However, lying uncomfortably full on the sofa for the rest of the evening, it doesn't take long for him to feel disappointed, angry, and disgusted with himself for losing control yet again.

Not all of our patients describe their difficulties with food in the same way as Angela and John. Leticia, for example, is certain her difficulty is that she just loves food "too much" and can't limit herself, especially if tempted by certain types of foods like carbohydrates.

Leticia's Story

Leticia had been following her "New Year's" diet, the latest in a lifelong series of diets, and was feeling dedicated to finally getting herself into shape. On this particular day, she was able to eat healthfully and moderately because she planned to go to her mother's home for a family get-together. She decided in advance that she would eat only tiny portions of her mother's specialties, but when she got to the house she found the aroma of the homemade food overwhelming. Once she took her first bite she was overcome with the desire to take a larger serving. Then, recognizing that she had broken her diet despite her resolve and all the hard work and exercise she had invested, she was filled with shame and disappointment. She thought to herself: "I've already blown it. The damage is done. I might as well binge all the way so I can start over tomorrow." She thus ate everything she wanted, including extra sweet potato pie. Initially, this resulted in an almost trancelike state in which all she focused on was the sensation of the food. Eventually she felt overly full and completely demoralized. At her next therapy session, when describing the episode, she didn't think she had been experiencing any identifiable emotions before she went to her mother's home and couldn't see how the DBT emotion regulation model applied to her.

We explained to Leticia that we had worked with many patients like her and agreed that the emotion that led her to binge was not present before she went to her mother's home.

A: Prompting event: the smell, sight, and taste of her mother's home cooking (see below).

B: Emotion: intense desire triggered by eating the food. Leticia experienced her desire as almost unbearable, because Leticia was apparently a *hedonic eater,* someone whose brain is wired to be highly sensitive to food with or without physical hunger (more on this below). Setting a limit or boundary with herself,

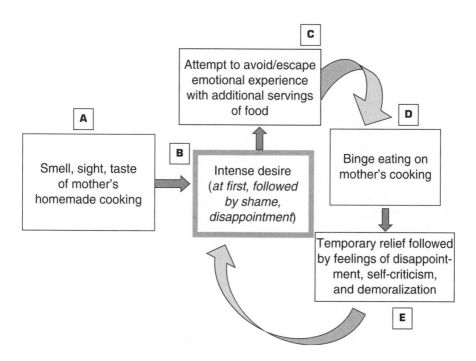

Leticia's DBT emotion regulation model for a binge.

especially after she had crossed the one she first set, felt emotionally impossible. This dynamic is explained by the DBT biosocial theory, which we will discuss later in this chapter in detail.

C: Breaking her diet triggered self-criticism, disappointment, and shame and led Leticia to put more food on her plate to try to avoid these emotions.

D: She then gave in to her urges and binged on everything she wanted to eat.

E: Temporarily this led to a reduction in her emotional discomfort, but in the long run it resulted in disappointment, self-criticism, and demoralization.

Leticia now understood desire to be the initial emotion she found so hard to tolerate, so the DBT emotion regulation model seemed to fit her experience. But if she couldn't blame herself and her lack of self-control, she could only blame her brain and biochemistry. Didn't that imply, she worried, that her situation was hopeless?

We don't believe that at all. We teach the DBT biosocial theory because, in our experience, it explains why some people have more difficulty tolerating emotional distress than others and it can help them be more compassionate and patient with themselves. If you recognize yourself as one of those people, you will understand just why the skills taught in this program will be so transformative for you.

We'll delve into the DBT biosocial theory in a minute, but first, think about whether the model of emotion regulation reflects your own experience with binge eating.

EXERCISE 1 Does the DBT Model of Emotion Regulation Fit Your Experience?

a. On a scale of 1–10, how well does the DBT emotion regulation model fit your binge eating or other problem eating behaviors?

| 1 | 2 | 3 | 4 | 5 | 6 | 7 | (8) | 9 | 10 |

Very poor fit · Perfect fit

b. Explain how the DBT emotion regulation model does or does not seem to explain your binge eating.

I do notice uncomfortable emotions

before emotional eating

What if you're not noticing any emotions (even desire) before bingeing? This program may help you uncover some by teaching you the skills to observe and describe your emotions more astutely.

What if you believe your binge eating is more like an addiction? We hope you'll work through this program anyway. Currently researchers can't say definitively whether food is truly an addictive substance, although we do know that some people appear to be genetically more vulnerable to binge eating carbohydrates and fats than others. Whatever your belief about binge eating and addiction, we've seen many people begin to eat foods in moderation that they once thought they were addicted to with the help of the skills in this book.

The DBT Biosocial Theory of Emotion Regulation

Angela's coworker may be provoked by the same boss but not find her emotions so intolerable that she feels she has to get rid of them no matter the cost to her in the long run. John finds it hard to tolerate feeling restless, annoyed, and possibly lonely where many others manage this discomfort. Leticia's brothers and sisters don't binge during the family get-together as she does. The DBT biosocial theory of emotion regulation helps to explain why some people may seem more vulnerable to experiencing strong emotions than others and why some people are more vulnerable to binge eating. Let's start with the biological (bio) part of the theory.

Biologically Based Emotional Vulnerability

How intensely we feel emotions lies on a spectrum, and this tendency is, in part, hard-wired or biological. Answering yes to one or more of the questions in the following quiz suggests that you may be high on the emotional vulnerability scale.

Emotional Vulnerability Quiz

1. Would you say you are more sensitive or more easily upset than others (whether or not you let others know what you're feeling)?

    (Yes)   No

2. Do you think you respond more intensely to your emotions than others (whether or not you express your emotions outwardly)?

    (Yes)   No

3. When you feel yourself become emotional or upset, do you tend to stay that way longer than others?

    Yes ⇨ No

Let's look more closely at what these three components of a biological vulnerability to emotion feel like:

1. *Sensitivity:* **It doesn't seem to take as much to trigger you.** A number of our patients have told us that for their whole lives they've been told they're "too sensitive."

2. *Intensity:* You tend to **react to a higher degree** than others in the same situation. People talk about "overreacting" to even the smallest hints of criticism or rejection. Even emotions that aren't expressed are felt more intensely than others describe.

3. *Duration:* You experience a **delayed return to "normal."** Your emotional reactions last longer, and sometimes you don't fully return to baseline before something else triggers an emotional reaction, only increasing your sensitivity and the likelihood that you'll get highly emotional.

If you're biologically vulnerable to emotion, you may describe yourself as emotionally thin-skinned. But what about the binge eater who feels like the opposite—*overly* emotionally controlled? This is not uncommon and actually makes a great deal of sense when you factor in years of using food or other behaviors to blunt or push away uncomfortable or threatening emotional experiences. Being overly controlled is still emotional dysregulation and can be improved with the skills in this book.

Biologically Based Vulnerability to Food and Its Rewarding Properties

People who binge might be biologically vulnerable not only to emotions but also to food and its rewarding properties. At this point, the research is not clear as to whether such vulnerabilities existed before the binge eating developed or were a result of binge eating, or if the two interacted over time, but we know that two factors are likely involved.

Hedonic eating, which seems to particularly affect Leticia, involves an increased appetite drive or preoccupation with highly desirable food even without physical hunger. It has been shown to be higher in people who binge eat. Individuals with high levels of hedonic hunger are particularly susceptible to food cues (e.g., the sight, smell, and taste of food) in the environment. Interestingly, the rewarding properties of food are "visible" in the brain before food is actually eaten. In other words, just anticipating food—how it will taste, how good it will feel to eat it, and how pleasurable eating will feel—cues the brain to react.

Importantly, there is evidence that the reward value of desirable foods is increased under distressing emotional states in binge eaters. In addition, research shows that repeatedly binge eating changes the brain's reward circuitry, so that the likelihood of overeating increases.

Delayed discounting refers to difficulty resisting short-term rewards (such as tempting binge foods) in favor of delayed or long-term goals. In other words, the value of future, or delayed, rewards is steeply discounted. This deficit, which affects Angela, John, and Leticia, is found more often among binge eaters than non-binge-eating obese or normal-weight individuals.

You may very well have a biological vulnerability to both emotions and food. However, that's not all that is usually involved in developing a pattern of binge eating to cope with uncomfortable emotions. The DBT biosocial theory refers to a biologically based sensitivity that interacted with the *environment* in which you were raised and specific life events you faced—the "social" part of biosocial.

Invalidating Environment

Some people binge eat due to a mismatch between their biological sensitivity and having experienced an emotionally invalidating environment. This environment could have been one you were raised in or are currently experiencing.

In an invalidating environment people respond inconsistently and/or inappropriately to your inner experiences (your thoughts, feelings, beliefs, and sensations) and oversimplify life's complexities. This doesn't mean that those who raised you didn't love you or didn't do the best they could to care for you. Maybe a parent taught you that emotions, particularly "negative" ones, were best unexpressed ("Stop crying or I'll give you something to cry about!") and you interpreted that message as meaning emotions shouldn't be felt. Or a parent encouraged you to set unrealistic goals with advice like "Smile and the world will smile with you." Instead of learning to expect mistakes and disappointments and value your ability to persist despite lack of immediate rewards when pursuing worthy goals, you became highly distressed by failure and quickly gave up. Just as the environment invalidated you, you learned to invalidate yourself.

John was an exuberant child who felt things intensely (a biological emotional vulnerability). When he was happy he was over-the-moon, and when something went wrong he suffered deeply. While the family had enough money, John's father was almost always working, leaving John in the care of his depressed mother. When his father *was* home, he seemed preoccupied and gruff. When something hurtful happened to John, he certainly wasn't given much attention from his mother, who usually ignored him or angrily told him to "Pull yourself together. You're absolutely fine." John was left with many overwhelming and painful emotions that felt intolerable to him. Being told he was "absolutely fine" by his mother confused him, because he didn't feel fine. On rare occasions when he hurt himself and cried or was sick, his mother would tell him to get a cookie from the kitchen.

Over time, John learned to soothe himself using food. He also learned to talk to himself in the same minimizing, invalidating way in which his mother spoke to him. For example, John learned to tell himself that nothing upsetting was taking place, despite being in situations in which he felt frustrated and lonely and feeling that something was missing from his life. As mentioned, he had difficulty identifying what he was feeling and mostly experienced himself as an unemotional person. He enjoyed the fact that people told him he seemed very in control, calm, and never seemed very affected by things that others reacted to. The truth was that, lacking emotional attunement, John had never learned skillful ways to tolerate or deal effectively with his negative emotional experiences. His parents had given him overly simplified ways of understanding the world. His goals for himself were often unrealistic, and when he couldn't reach them, he became extremely distressed.

Does any of John's experience sound familiar? Patients often tell us that as children there was little to no room for their emotions, especially negative ones such as anger or intense sadness. Maybe you were taught to ignore your real feelings, and if you couldn't you faced the danger of not being liked or of feeling like an imposition or a burden. Or maybe you were being mistreated and felt responsible and fearful of calling attention to yourself. Often patients will describe learning to override their food satiation signals, for example, if they were encouraged to eat past the point of fullness: "There are starving kids in China" or "I went to all this effort to make you a nice meal."

As mentioned, invalidating environments also exist (or can continue) in adulthood. Perhaps your partner shows discomfort with some of your feelings or thoughts but not others, and you're never sure what kind of reaction you're going to get, so you've started to tell yourself you're not even *having* these inner experiences. As a result, you may have never learned healthy ways to cope with your emotions, particularly distressing ones, or you've started suppressing them.

Angela generally took on most of the household and child-rearing responsibilities because her husband spent his time at home on his own interests, claiming his job was so demanding that he had a right to his free time. When she tried to ask for help or express unhappiness, she was criticized for acting like a nag.

An invalidating environment can leave highly emotionally vulnerable individuals with difficulty tolerating distress and/or difficulty believing that their emotional responses are accurate interpretations of events. They also have a tendency to look outside themselves for cues about how they are feeling. For example, Angela, wanting to keep her marriage peaceful, learned to keep quiet about her unhappiness and resentment. She tried to do this at work as well. When she had difficulty with her boss, Angela blamed herself and told herself to get over it, that she was too sensitive. Food was one of the few things in her life that didn't expect anything from her and didn't criticize her.

What about Culture?

Leticia feels that she wasn't raised in an invalidating environment, although she does have the vulnerability factors of being a hedonic eater and having poor tolerance for intense emotions, especially emotions such as desire. But significantly, Leticia was raised in a culture where food is celebratory and synonymous with love and family. She commented that not partaking in the celebration would make her feel left out and disconnected from her family. Food plays an important role in many cultures, and how it played a role in your family or culture may be an important factor to consider.

Having a Stick Shift in an Automatic Transmission World

You may be coming to the realization that you're not like those people who seem to "just eat normally" or to be able to control themselves around food. One way to think about it is to imagine yourself as a stick-shift transmission living in a world of automatic transmissions. You may have been trying to operate without knowing how the gears work. Learning to drive a stick shift initially requires paying more attention to the mechanics of driving—at least until you get the hang of it. This program will help you personalize your own operating manual so you can stop stalling out.

This may be hard to accept. Just thinking about these issues and working to change problematic patterns will likely bring up painful emotional experiences. Courage is required to face the discomfort that is likely to arise as we ask you to consider giving up food, the very thing that can make you feel better (at least in the short term). But don't worry—later chapters in this program will focus on increasing your ability to regulate your emotions without using food.

Chapter 1 Summary

As the DBT biosocial theory suggests, you may have a biological vulnerability to emotions that has interacted with sustained invalidation of your emotional experience. The DBT emotion regulation model shows that turning to food does, *temporarily*, decrease your distress, by providing an escape from intense and uncomfortable emotions. In the long run, however, binge eating increases your guilt, despair, and shame and hence makes you even more vulnerable to binge eating. We have found that when our patients understand how these models explain their binge eating, they more easily let go of some of the harsh judgment of their own behaviors and feel more motivated and prepared to learn new skills to manage their discomfort instead of turning to food.

Homework

We mentioned in the Introduction that the exercises and homework assignments in this book are based on those used in our research studies. Patients who worked through them were the ones most likely to successfully stop binge eating. If you have difficulty attempting them and have a therapist, make sure to bring this up! And if you don't have a therapist, strongly consider getting one or checking in with a trusted friend.

Complete the exercises below, including checking the boxes when you have finished. You'll be accumulating skills throughout this program, and checking off the boxes at the end of each chapter helps you stay accountable—to say nothing of giving you a sense of accomplishment and happiness. If you need more than one week to finish a chapter, you can indicate you've completed the weekly homework assignments more than once by adding another check mark either inside or next to these boxes.

HOMEWORK EXERCISE 1-A

Filling In the DBT Emotion Regulation Model for an Episode of Binge Eating

Let's look at a typical binge for you to see if it fits with the DBT emotion regulation model. Describe your most recent binge or problem eating episode below. When did it take place? Where were you?

Had to write grant proposal - Dont want to.

Anger

_____

_____

_____

_____

_____

What was the prompting event or environmental trigger that might have led to this binge? Write that in box A at the far left of the diagram on the facing page. (Perhaps it was being criticized or receiving a compliment, attending a social event, being given a new responsibility at work, coming home to an empty house, etc.). It's OK if you're not sure—just do your best.

What emotions were you feeling because of the trigger? Enter those emotions (e.g., anxiety, anger, shame, irritation, sadness, worry, relief, happiness, pleasure, guilt) in box B. Again, just do your best to identify what you can.

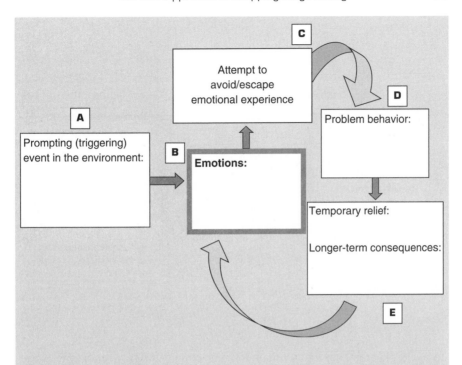

We've filled in box C for you—that you attempted to avoid experiencing the uncomfortable emotions.

What, specifically, did you do? Did you binge, binge and purge, emotionally eat, overeat? Fill in the behavior you did in box D.

What were the immediate consequences of the binge (or other problem behavior)? Did you feel better temporarily? Describe this in box E. What were the longer-term consequences? Describe this in box E as well.

Here is how one of our patients, Kat, filled this out:

My most recent binge episode was last night. I had had two days of really bad allergy symptoms, including itchy eyes, hives on my eyelids, sneezing, and an overall sense of physical discomfort. I happened to glance in the mirror as I passed the bathroom, and I was revolted by my appearance. At my worst, which this was, I feel like I look like the Quaker Oats man—fat, ruddy-faced, and old.

I was home with my husband watching a movie, and I went upstairs and took a little box of chocolate truffles out of the fridge and absolutely knew that I was going to eat all of them. There were about a dozen. Somehow, I managed to offer some to Tom—probably to pretend to myself that I wasn't really bingeing. He ate two or three, and I ate all the rest.

In the diagram on page 34, Kat wrote that the prompting event (A) was catching a glimpse of herself in the mirror. This triggered emotions she recorded in (B) as disgust, self-loathing, rage, fear, and sadness. She then attempted

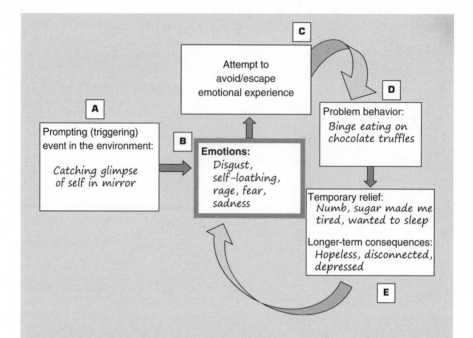

to avoid experiencing these uncomfortable emotions (C) by turning to binge eating on the box of chocolate truffles (D). The immediate consequences she wrote in (E) included feeling numb, feeling tired due to the sugar, and wanting to sleep. She described the longer-term consequences of the binge as feeling hopeless, disconnected, and even more depressed.

❑ I have completed the exercise using a recent binge episode.

HOMEWORK EXERCISE 1-B

Reactions to Learning about the DBT Emotion Regulation Model
and Biosocial Theory

We've heard from patients that once they've learned about the DBT emotion regulation model and the biosocial theory their "eyes have been opened and there is no going back." What does that mean to you in terms of being more aware of connections between your emotions and urges to binge or overeat? Do you notice yourself being more aware of your sensitivity to your emotions? What are your recollections about experiencing any emotional invalidation growing up and/or in your current environment? Use the space below to answer.

_____

_____

_____

_____

_____

_____

_____

_____

_____

_____

_____

Kat wrote:

I have been more aware of my emotional reactions and responses. It mostly brings up for me reminders of how devastated I was this last year when I discovered Tom was having an affair.

This discovery was a terrible blow to my self-esteem and to my belief in my marriage and my relationship with Tom. I've never experienced such a deep sense of loss.

I also felt like an ugly, old, neutered woman who has outlived her use and should have been put out to sea on an iceberg (if there are any left) to just drift away.

I think that rage and grief have equal valence and that just knowing this may be able to help me short-circuit a binge.

HOMEWORK EXERCISE 1-C

Being More Aware of Your Emotions and Their Connections
to Binge Eating This Coming Week and Beyond

Take a moment to think about the DBT emotion regulation model and the bio-social theory every day this coming week (especially after episodes of binge eating, if any). What does it bring up for you when you become more aware of your emotions and how they connect to your binge eating? How do you think your new awareness about your vulnerability to binge eating might help you in the weeks to come?

_____

_____

_____

_____

_____

_____

_____

_____

_____

_____

_____

_____

_____

_____

_____

_____

Kat wrote:

Growing up, my father would rage and was unpredictably violent. It ter-rified me. I never knew what would set him off and tried to draw as little attention as I could so as to avoid making him angry. So I'm realizing I never had a healthy model of anger and never learned how to deal with it in others or in myself. I always felt that being too angry was a problem instead of realizing that it wasn't anger itself, it's the way a person behaves in response to anger that's the problem. My father threw things and I try to stuff anger down with food or in the past sometimes didn't eat enough. Thinking about my childhood helps me recognize how difficult it has been this past year to tolerate my fury at my husband. No wonder I've craved so much chocolate and everything else I could find to feel numb. Taking time to be aware of this connection every day and why anger is especially hard for me to tolerate is a very helpful reminder to not repeat old patterns.

❑ I have paid attention to (tried to notice) the influence of learning about the emotion regulation model and biosocial theory every day this week (espe-cially after episodes of binge eating, if any).

2

Making a Commitment
to Stop Binge Eating

In this chapter we are going to do less of the "talking" and instead will lead you through a number of exercises to help you reflect deeply on why you want to stop binge eating. Of course you want to stop or you wouldn't be reading this. But our experience has taught us that most difficult-to-change behaviors, like binge eating, serve very important purposes for us. Understanding these is a crucial step in stopping these behaviors for good.

Having to face the negative impact that binge eating has had on your life may make these exercises painful. Often we remind our patients of what you likely already know: Being willing to look back at how you got to where you are now is a vital step in learning how to get to where you want to go.

The time you spend on the exercises in this chapter will be well spent. Exploring your complex relationship with food as well as your commitment to changing that relationship forms an invaluable basis for the rest of your work in this program. If you find yourself struggling in the coming weeks and months (which, by the way, is normal!), you'll likely find your responses in this chapter remind you what led you to this program and give you the motivation you're looking for to stick with it despite temporary challenges.

Learning from the Past

EXERCISE 1 Looking at Your Attempts to Stop Binge Eating

John had tried multiple times to stop binge eating and initially was convinced that he simply lacked willpower, that he was a failure, that his binge eating was an impossible habit to break. After working through some of his binge episodes using the emotion regulation model and learning about the biosocial theory, he began to understand there were good reasons he had had so much difficulty stopping binge eating in the past despite trying multiple diets and diet pills from his doctor. A top reason was that there were too many tempting foods in his house. He hadn't understood how emotionally vulnerable he was, especially late at night or on the weekends, and how he didn't know how to tolerate feelings like annoyance and loneliness. It was just too easy to turn to those foods and binge when he didn't have any healthy ways to cope. A second reason, he saw, was that he simply had never made any time on a regular basis to reduce his considerable level of stress. He'd never been willing to put time into regular physical activity, for instance. A third reason was that his weekends were largely unstructured. He realized he had set himself up to fail because his relentless focus on work and lack of priority placed on friendships left him often feeling isolated and lonely.

a. **What have you tried, and why hasn't it worked?** We assume that picking up this book was probably not your first attempt to gain control over your eating. Take a moment to think about things you've done to try to stop binge eating in the past and reasons those attempts did not work. Write down the top three reasons below.

1. _____

_____

_____

_____

_____

2. _____

_____

_____

_____

3. _____

_____

_____

_____

_____

Below is an example of how Kat, introduced in Chapter 1, completed this exercise:

1. *I tried to use "all or nothing," black/white behaviors. I would more or less starve myself for a day or two and then totally lose control and binge for the following week or more.*

2. *I was too ashamed to get help, and my bingeing was a secret. I've never been really overweight, so it was easy to hide the fact that I had a binge-eating disorder from the rest of the world and also from myself to a certain degree.*

3. *I was focused on what the scale read. I was motivated by numbers and dress sizes—not by physical and emotional health.*

b. **What helped you stop binge eating (even temporarily)?** Now we'd like you to think about times when you've had periods of success at controlling your binge eating. *Whether or not these periods were followed by a return to binge eating, periods with reduced binge eating are successes.* What are the top three factors that contributed to these successes? Write your answers below. If you need more room, use an extra sheet of paper.

  If you are having difficulty answering this question, perhaps it would help to think about times when you've been able to stop yourself from binge eating despite experiencing urges or cravings. What factors (e.g., making time for self-care such as meditation, exercise, or journaling; having some structure around mealtimes) helped? You might also take a look at how Kat answered (on the next page), to see if that prompts your thinking.

1. _____

   _____

   _____

   _____

   _____

   _____

   _____

   _____

2. _____

   _____

   _____

_____

_____

_____

_____

3. _____

_____

_____

_____

_____

_____

Kat wrote:

1. I'm not actually sure I've ever been able to stop myself from binge-ing due to my own conscious efforts. The absence of binge eating has primarily been the result of external factors that affected my moods. For instance, I was binge free 1 month when I was on vacation and living with my mother. It was a very peaceful month with my father away when we were staying at a cottage near a lake. I remember eating fresh foods, taking long walks, and having very few if any struggles with binge eating. Another time I was binge free was during the first year or so that my husband and I were together. I think that I was on a high from being with someone I was crazy about and I had no or very little impulse to binge. It wasn't a struggle.

2. My binge eating started when I was really young, before age 10. It went away for a period when I was 11 and I came home to find out my parents had returned my dog to the breeder. My dog had bitten me, so it wasn't a surprise that it was going to happen; I just didn't know when. But when I came home and he was gone, it was a shock and I fell into a deep, quiet depression that lasted a year—till I was 12. I had no appetite, and grief dominated any other feelings. My binge eating has mostly been triggered by anxiety, anger, or rejection. But with real and deep sadness or grief I had no desire to binge.

3. *What I'm most aware of in writing these answers is that control-ling my binge eating has been dependent on external circumstances, just as bingeing has. I didn't use any particular tools to keep from bingeing. The environment changed, and that interfered with most opportunities to binge. Things like having a stressful or less stress-ful job, or times when I joined Weight Watchers and ate in a more structured way.*

c. **What factors have influenced your binge eating?** Take a moment to see if you can figure out some of the factors that influence *your* binge eating by reviewing your answers to **a** and **b,** above. Do certain triggers consistently lead to binge eating, or do they do so only under certain circumstances? Maybe at other times you have been able to find a different way to cope with a strong emotion instead of turning to binge eating?

Angela was able to put the information from **a** and **b** together to see a pat-tern—she binges far more often during the week than on the weekend. The triggers for her binges, at least her most intense binges, seem to be interac-tions at work, usually with her boss. She realizes that she has less difficulty controlling her urges to binge when her boss is away on vacation or when she herself is away. She also has more control over her eating when she's involved with activities that are not related to work or home and provide a break between her two areas of greatest involvement. For example, she had a period of successful eating during the time she was taking a yoga class with friends right after work instead of going straight home or when she and her husband went for a walk immediately after dinner.

Use the space below to discuss the factors that influence your binge eating and write about any patterns you notice.

_____

_____

_____

_____

_____

_____

_____

_____

_____

_____

_____

_____

Kat wrote:

It's pretty obvious to me that my binge eating is always triggered by some relational conflict. There are two things I'm aware of that help me manage impulses to binge. The first and most important is having a witness—my therapist, close friend, physician—someone who sees and understands the struggle and who can tolerate my discomfort without taking it on.

   The second is thinking about my future self. It's sort of like remembering something that hasn't happened yet, combined with memories of real past events. For example, I might imagine feeling comfortable in a dress I really like, or singing with my friends and thinking about the music and not about how I look while I'm singing!

We would like you to build an understanding of why you binge. Binges may feel random, but they actually occur under particular circumstances for specific reasons. The process of recovery involves discovering the reasons binges occur, which will allow you to make the changes you need to stop them from continuing to take place.

Examining the Present: Evaluating Pros/Cons of Binge Eating

EXERCISE 2   Identifying the Advantages and Disadvantages of Binge Eating

At this point in the program we ask our patients, as we will now be asking you, to look at the pros and cons of binge eating. Clearly binge eating is something you want to stop; that is the aim of this program. But it's important to acknowledge the advantages that binge eating *has had for you*. Some of our patients can readily acknowledge these "pros," whereas others say there are no advantages, that binge eating is purely a negative experience. Even if you feel that is true, we've listed some advantages patients have mentioned to us and ask you to review them to see if any are true for you or if they prompt you to think of others. Write your own advantages in the space following the examples.

- "Eating is one of the main ways I can feel good. It's one of my only rewards or treats."

- "It's an escape. It comforts and calms me."

- "I enjoy food and I deserve to eat as much as I want to, when I want to."

- "Food is something that only I can control—no one is going to tell me I can't have it."

- "Binge eating gives me a feeling of distance from problems I don't know how to solve. It's like a time-out."

- "Food is a big part of how my family shows affection and celebrates."

- "Binge eating and being overweight give me an excuse to avoid things."

- "I am so stressed out from my day that eating calms me down so I can relax or sleep."

- "Binge eating lets me expect less from myself so that I don't have to feel the discomfort of trying new things and can therefore avoid feeling disappointment."

Top advantages of binge eating:

- _____
  _____
  _____
  _____

- _____
  _____
  _____
  _____

- _____
  _____
  _____
  _____

- _____
  _____
  _____
  _____

- _____
  _____
  _____

● _____
   _____
   _____
   _____

● _____
   _____
   _____
   _____
   _____

● _____
   _____
   _____
   _____

● _____
   _____
   _____
   _____

● _____
   _____
   _____
   _____

Kat wrote:

- Binge eating helps me avoid feeling the pain of my troubled marriage.

- Binge eating allows me to expect less of myself so that I don't reach as high. I preempt failure.

- Binge eating in the moment gives me a break from my concerns about my health, including my high blood sugar.

- Binge eating distracts me from anxiety-provoking challenges, like auditioning or singing performances.

The previously cited advantages don't paint the whole picture. As you well know, there are serious disadvantages to binge eating. Think of the top disadvantages of binge eating for you and list them below. Again, we've started you off with a few possibilities.

- "Binge eating feels embarrassing and shameful."

- "Binge eating makes me feel wild and out of control."

- "Binge eating causes me to avoid things that could make my life richer and more meaningful. I lose my desire to be with others, and I just want to isolate myself."

- "Binge eating harms my physical health (e.g., weight, cholesterol, blood pressure, joints)."

- "Binge eating makes me not like or respect myself."

- "Binge eating tricks me into thinking my needs are being met when they're not."

- "Binge eating damages my self-esteem."

- "Binge eating makes me feel intense guilt and overwhelming regret."

- "Binge eating makes me secretive. I don't want to completely let others in and have them find out about this part of me."

- "Binge eating prevents me from being fully happy and satisfied with myself."

- _____
  _____
  _____

- _____
  _____
  _____

- _____
  _____
  _____

- _____
  _____
  _____

- _____
  _____
  _____

- _____
  _____
  _____

- _____
  _____
  _____

- _____
  _____
  _____

- _____
  _____
  _____

Kat wrote:

- *Binge eating makes me feel guilty and ashamed and hate myself.*

- *Binge eating makes me afraid of food.*

- *Binge eating makes me feel like hiding, and I'm tired of hiding.*

- *Binge eating makes me physically uncomfortable, which makes it harder to feel attractive.*

- *Binge eating makes me feel hopeless about the future.*

- *Binge eating lowers my self-esteem, leading me to stay in my comfort zone and not challenge myself to be creative and take risks.*

- *Binge eating scares me because I know I'm contributing to my high blood sugar.*

EXERCISE 3   Comparing the Advantages and Disadvantages
of Binge Eating

Look over and compare your two lists of the top advantages and disadvantages of binge eating in Exercise 2. The advantages look compelling, don't they? Binge eating is immediately gratifying and so powerful that it allows you, temporarily at least, to ignore the painful longer-term disadvantages.

It's important to ask yourself if continuing to binge eat would be incompatible with leading a happy, highly satisfying life. Could you have both? If you're thinking maybe you could, remember that when we refer to a "happy, highly satisfying life," we're not talking about a life in which you are simply existing or "getting through" and trying to minimize pain. You may already have that.

We're talking about feeling fully alive, as though you are living up to your potential. We are talking about having the best life that you are capable of.

Are you able to convince yourself that continuing to binge eat is incompatible with your living a happy, highly satisfying life? Write your thoughts below.

_____

_____

_____

_____

_____

_____

_____

_____

_____

Kat wrote:

Uh . . . Yeah. I'm totally convinced. I've got too much that I want to do and have no idea how much longer I'll have on Planet Earth. I absolutely know that I don't want to spend whatever time I have left to me dealing with bingeing!!!

EXERCISE 4 Identifying Your Values

We now ask you to turn your attention to the values that are most important to you. By values, we mean your principles or standards of behavior, what you judge as important in life. Below we have included examples of *some* values that people may hold.* If your most important values are not on the list, please add your own. At the end of the list we will ask you to choose the five values you believe best represent you. Example values:

Achievement: to accomplish important goals

Authority: to be in charge and responsible for others

Adventure: to have new and exciting adventures

Autonomy: to be self-determined and independent

---

*Adapted from *Personal Values Card Sort* by William R. Miller, Janet C'de Baca, Daniel B. Matthews, and Paula L. Wilbourne (2001). Albuquerque: University of New Mexico. Public domain.

Beauty: to appreciate (and create) beauty

Challenge: to take on difficult tasks and problems

Change: to have a variety of life experiences

Comfort: to have a pleasant and comfortable life

Contribution: to make a lasting contribution in the world

Creativity: to engage in creative expression

Duty: to carry out duty and obligations

Empathy: the ability to understand and share the feelings of another

Fairness: the just treatment of others

Family: to have a happy, loving family

Forgiveness: to be forgiving of myself and others

Friendship: to have close, supportive relationships

Fun: to play and have fun

Growth: to keep developing and growing

Health: to be physically healthy

Honesty: to be honest and truthful

Hope: to maintain a positive and optimistic outlook

Inner Peace: to experience personal peace

Knowledge: to learn and contribute valuable ideas

Love: to love and be loved by those close to me

Moderation: to avoid excess and find balance

Nonconformity: to question and challenge authority and norms

Nurturance: to take care of and nurture others

Rationality: to be guided by reason and logic

Romance: to have intense, exciting love in my life

Safety: to be safe and secure

Self-acceptance: to accept myself as I am with self-compassion

Self-control: to be disciplined in my own actions

Spirituality: to grow and mature spiritually

_____

_____

_____

_____

a. **Pick the top five values that you believe best represent you and list them below.**

1. _____

2. _____

3. _____

4. _____

5. _____

Kat listed the following values, two of which she added (Authenticity, Wisdom):

1. *Creativity*

2. *Self-acceptance*

3. *Growth*

4. *Wisdom—being able to see beneath the superficial to what matters deeply and to act upon that knowledge*

5. *Authenticity—being genuine, truthful, not pretending to be anyone but myself*

b. **For each of your top five values, write down what that value means to you personally and what helps you know that it is important to you.** For example, have you made any decisions or taken any actions based on that value?

1. _____

_____

_____

_____

2. _____

_____

_____

_____

_____

3. _____

_____

_____

_____

4. _____

_____

_____

_____

5. _____

_____

_____

_____

Kat wrote:

1. *Creativity feels like the basis of who I am, the best part of me, the part that allows me to feel like an artist and most alive. Because I value creativity so much, it has influenced my decisions about my profession.*

2. *Self-acceptance—when I feel most centered, I am accepting of myself and feel compassionate toward myself. This allows me to feel accepting and compassionate of others too.*

3. *Growth is important to me so that I feel stimulated as a person and that I am learning and developing and taking advantage of being alive.*

4. *Wisdom—I admire people I consider wise, and I want to be like them, focusing my life on the things that really matter instead of wasting time on superficial issues.*

5. *Authenticity—I value letting myself be seen as I truly am instead of hiding or trying to impress others.*

c. **How is your binge eating connected to each value?** Does binge eating help or interfere with each value? Describe the connection you see between your binge eating and your ability to live out each of your core values.

1. _____

_____

_____

_____

_____

2. _____

_____

_____

_____

_____

3. _____

_____

_____

_____

_____

4. _____

_____

_____

_____

_____

5. _____

_____

_____

_____

_____

Kat wrote:

1. *Binge eating is in direct opposition to everything I value most. When I binge, it interferes with my feeling that I have the right to be creative. I feel like I'm an imposter because none of my fellow artists would behave like I do.*

2. *Binge eating makes me hate myself. Without compassion, I can't hold on to self-acceptance.*

3. *Binge eating causes me to hide. It saps me of energy and vitality. I lose interest in growing and learning. It feels like all I can do is try to*

> *trudge through another day so I can get into bed. I lose my goals for more.*
>
> 4. *Binge eating narrows my focus and fills me with self-loathing. I'm so trapped in my own head that I don't have the self-acceptance I need to truly take risks and grow—so I don't have the characteristics that are essential to gain wisdom.*
>
> 5. *Because I'm so ashamed of my binge eating, I keep it inside as a private, ugly secret. This prevents me from being authentic. I even lie to myself, rationalizing doing things that I know set me up to binge.*

The purpose of this exercise was to see whether or not you feel your binge eating is consistent with your core values. Most often, people find there is a huge disconnect between their values and binge eating. If that's the case for you, it gives you all the more reason to stop binge eating!

Looking to the Future: A Life Free of Binge Eating

The following exercise is designed to get you thinking about what a life free of binge eating would look like.

EXERCISE 5 What Would Your Life Be Like without Binge Eating?

a. **If you were to gaze into a crystal ball and see yourself after you stopped binge eating, what sorts of things would you see yourself doing?** What would your life be like? How would it be different from your current life? For example, what might be the impact on your health in terms of your energy level, the activities you're involved in, the style of clothes you choose? If you've been binge eating so long that it feels hard to imagine your future without binge eating, try to focus on the shorter-term consequences you'd experience. For example, what would your mornings feel like if you hadn't binged the evening before? How would your finances be affected if you weren't spending so much on binge foods?

_____

_____

_____

_____

_____

_____

_____

_____

_____

Kat wrote:

I would feel . . . No . . . I WILL feel comfortable in my body. I'll have greater self-compassion with which to engage in activities I love, like singing, as well as activities I hate—like balancing my checkbook—no more checkbook binges! I won't harshly judge my appearance because I'll be too busy doing other things! And I'll actually enjoy eating and sharing meals with people I love!

b. **What did you notice most about your future life without binge eating?** What do you think about the differences between this future self and your current reality? Please discuss below.

_____

_____

_____

_____

_____

_____

_____

Kat wrote:

I discovered that I enjoy eating! I think I spend so much time feeling that food is a threat that I haven't really thought much about how it could become a pleasure. When I'm not a binge-crazed loony-tunes, I enjoy cooking and preparing food for other people. This is really something to look forward to! I know how pleasurable it is to actually feel hungry and then eat. And if I'm not bingeing, I'll have the opportunity to do this three times a day.

Making a Commitment

You may not be convinced that stopping binge eating is right for you at this moment. This decision is obviously completely up to you. The exercises above may have revealed that binge eating is not really interfering in a major way with your quality of life. Many people accept eating as they want to and are able to feel extremely good about themselves. If that describes you, you have discovered something very important about yourself. If this situation changes in the future, know that this program is here for you.

It's also possible, given your current circumstances, that the advantages of binge eating outweigh the disadvantages. Right now, you're willing to accept these disadvantages (e.g., lowered self-esteem, health problems, and/or using food to avoid or numb yourself to emotionally challenging situations) even if you don't like them. This is something only you can decide.

That being said, it is also important to ask yourself whether you are minimizing the harm associated with binge eating because stopping seems too daunting. This program has helped many people, and there is no reason it can't help you. If you have checked in with yourself and still believe that stopping binge eating isn't right for you right now, that is important for you to know. Again, if the situation changes, know that this program is here for you.

You're still reading! So we assume you've made the decision to stop binge eating and give yourself a chance to live the life you want to lead, and that cessation of bingeing is the only sane thing to do.

Research has shown that there is power in making a commitment—a power that isn't present from simply saying "I'll try." Studies have demonstrated that people who make a commitment, either verbally or by signing their names, are more likely to follow through. Saying "I'll try my best" leaves the door open, even if only just a crack, for turning to binge eating. In a sense, trying is saying "75% of me will be on board, but if it gets really bad, I'm going to give myself the option to go back to binge eating." It's actually in that 25% of the time that reminding yourself of your absolute commitment to *no* binge eating will make it much more likely you will make it through without turning to food. Making a commitment, which is based on your having fully examined how stopping binge eating is connected to your life's goals and values, means you don't have to rethink it when you're in a stressful situation and the "pros" of binge eating feel compelling. You've decided what is in your long-term best interests, and it doesn't include binge eating. But don't worry, we are not asking you to make this commitment with nothing else to support you. We are simply asking you to commit to turning to this program first. By committing to turning to the program in this book, instead of turning straight to food, you are giving yourself a chance to make necessary changes using the

Concerns about Making a Commitment

Concern: How can I make the commitment if I'm not sure I can keep it?

Response: Are you worried about turning to food (and not the skills in the program) right now? Or are you worried you won't turn to the skills in the program in the future? We are talking about **this one moment, right now.** Not about the future. After all, life is made up of one moment at a time, a continuous set of present moments. Can you make a commitment to stop binge eating and turn to the skills in the program instead of food in this one moment, right now? If so, just start with that.

Concern: How can I keep this commitment when it is impossible for me not to go straight to eating food?

Response: Would it literally be **impossible?** We know it would likely be very, very difficult, uncomfortable, and scary to think of living your life without immediately using food as a means of comfort. But are you saying that you think there is no way for you to **physically survive** turning to the program before turning to food? We argue, and you would have to agree, you **could** survive by turning to the program first. Please don't let the fear of the future paralyze you. We believe that you can do this. We would not ask you to do anything we knew was not possible. You *can* do it.

Concern: It might be **possible,** but I certainly wouldn't be able to. I'm certain I would fail!

Response: Perhaps it feels less risky to predict your failure to stop bingeing than it would be to commit to this program only to fail at it. We understand this kind of thinking. Yet we know from research on commitments that when people don't make a commitment or say they will accept less—when, right from the beginning, they say there's no hope—the likelihood of success is lowered.

Concern: What if life without binge eating isn't possible?

Response: Many people with binge-eating disorders become so accustomed to a lower quality of life that it can begin to feel as if nothing more is possible. We are asking you to envision having a life that may indeed seem out of reach, one that may feel as if it is too much for you to want for yourself. *It **is** scary, but we believe you can do it. We believe you can let yourself want your life to be that good.*

Concern: It feels like just making the commitment sets me up to binge!

Response: You're worried about committing—you think that if you do you're setting yourself up for failure, that you'd commit here and then go straight out to binge. One thing that might be helpful to ask yourself: *"Is it possible to have a goal while knowing that you may not be able to meet it? Does falling short of it make it wrong to have the goal in the first place?"*

healthy coping skills we are teaching you to manage the emotional distress that underlies your binge eating.

To recap, we are asking you to make a commitment to:

STOP BINGE EATING
and
TURN TO THIS PROGRAM FIRST!

Before making this commitment, take a moment.

Do you have any concerns?

In the box on page 55 are concerns we've heard from patients in the past, some of which you may share, and how we've responded to them.

Look over what you've written so far. Breathe. How is this sitting with you? This is a serious commitment. Check deep within yourself. If you need to, look over your argument convincing yourself about the incompatibility of binge eating and living a highly satisfying life.

Remember John? Like many people, he struggled with signing the commitment. John worked in finance and was used to things being black and white, right or wrong. He had completed all the exercises in this chapter except for the last one, but he didn't feel he could sign the commitment to stop binge eating because he could not predict what the future would hold and he hadn't yet learned any of the skills in the rest of the book. Further, holding himself to his commitments was an important value of his, and the possibility of not being able to meet the commitment was anxiety provoking.

This struggle demonstrates how powerful making commitments can be! Although the skills in the rest of this book will help you stop binge eating, we feel strongly that once you have decided to stop, and are actively working on doing so, you may surprise yourself with what new strategies you come up with on your own. When this point was discussed with John and he was reminded that he was making a commitment in *this moment, based on right now and not the future,* he was able to sign the commitment agreement. Once John made the commitment he poured his strength into the program, with great results.

EXERCISE 6 Writing Out Your Commitment to Stop Binge Eating

When you are ready, in your own words, write your commitment to yourself to stop binge eating (or engaging in other problem eating behaviors) and to **turn to this program *first* instead of turning to food as a way of coping with emotional distress.**

_____

_____

_____

_____

_____

_____

_____

_____

_____

_____

_____

_____

_____

_____

_____

Signed: _____ Date: _____

Kat wrote:

In order to honor the value of my life, binge eating is NOT an option. When I turn to binge eating, I'm not really living. I'm choosing to cut off having access to my emotions and instead am choosing to numb myself. It is a vote of no confidence in myself and my ability to face reality and grow. I want to know who I truly am before I die. Binge eating is denying difficult feelings and pretending to be fine. But I want to be truly alive, even if that means experiencing pain and rage and sadness. Turning to this program before I turn to food means giving myself a chance to use healthy skills to cope with my feelings—which it's time I learned! I want more self-love, self-compassion, and self-respect. I want to use my feelings in my art and be wiser as a person. The oblivion of binge eating is a short-term solution but a long-term waste of my opportunities on this planet. Not to mention the health consequences and the effects on my body. I deserve more!

Congratulations!!!

Now that you've made a commitment to stopping binge eating and turning to this program first, we can dive into the details in the following chapters.

Chapter 2 Summary

Throughout this chapter we have asked you to think hard about binge eating and to consider whether you can live your life to the fullest *and* binge eat. Because you are still reading, we assume you've decided there is not room for both.

We have asked you about how your past history of binge eating is related to the DBT emotion regulation model of binge eating. We've also asked you to look at the impact that binge eating currently has on your life and whether your core values are consistent with binge eating. Finally, we've asked you to think about what life will be like without binge eating.

Even though working through this chapter may have been difficult, we hope you are finishing with a sense of excitement about the future. It's OK to be both scared and excited at the same time—that's completely understandable. In the next chapter we will look at how the program is set up and introduce you to an important tool that you will use throughout this treatment.

Homework

Complete the following exercises, including checking the boxes after completing each assignment.

> **HOMEWORK EXERCISE 2-A**
> Creating a Wallet-Sized Pros/Cons of Binge Eating Card
>
> For this exercise, use a 3" × 5" index card or any other sheet of paper that can be folded to fit into a wallet or purse.
>
> On one side of this card, **list the five worst consequences of continuing binge eating.** On the other side, **list the five most positive consequences of stopping binge eating.** Put this card in your wallet, purse, or another place that is easily accessible so that you can quickly refer to it when you need it. Some of our patients have found it helpful to use their smartphones, such as by typing in a copy of their consequences and/or storing a picture of their card.
>
> **For Kat,** the five worst consequences of continuing to binge eat were:
>
> 1. Self-hatred
>
> 2. Depression

3. Health problems

4. Lack of creativity

5. Inauthenticity

For Kat, the top five positive consequences of stopping binge eating were:

1. Will have energy to live my life with authenticity, find out who I really am instead of wasting time hating myself or being numb

2. Feel greater self-acceptance, self-confidence, self-love

3. Won't feel like I have this big secret I'm always hiding, more room for creativity and growth

4. Will be more comfortable in my body

5. Better physical health

❏ I have filled out a Pros/Cons of Binge Eating Card listing the consequences of binge eating and of stopping binge eating.

HOMEWORK EXERCISE 2-B
Creating a Commitment Card

On another 3" × 5" index card or other piece of paper, copy some or all (depending on space) of what you stated as your commitment to stop binge eating **and turn to this program first, instead of turning to food, as a way of coping with emotional distress.** You may also wish to copy this onto your smartphone.

On her Commitment Card, Kat wrote:

In order to honor the value of my life, binge eating is NOT an option. When I turn to binge eating, I'm not really living. I want to know who I truly am before I die. Binge eating is denying difficult feelings so I can make it through my life and not create waves. But I want to be truly alive, even if that means experiencing difficult feelings. The oblivion of binge eating, though tempting in the short run, is ultimately a heartbreaking waste of my opportunity to live fully and authentically.

❏ I have created a Commitment Card (that I can carry with me) to remind me that I am committed to stopping binge eating and turning to the program as opposed to turning to food.

HOMEWORK EXERCISE 2-C
Creating a Motivation Card

If there was anything that particularly struck you while reading the chapter that you think will help with your motivation, copy that down on a 3" × 5" index card or foldable piece of paper you can carry with you so you can remind yourself of it.

This too may be valuable to copy onto your smartphone. You can leave space so you can add to this card during the program.

Kat wrote on her Motivation Card:

Sometimes I might need a witness to help me keep from getting lost, to help me keep to this program and my commitment. This is so important because the oblivion binge eating offers can be tempting. My values are too important to lose sight of.

❑ I have made a Motivation Card with my notes of anything else from this chapter that will help keep me motivated.

HOMEWORK EXERCISE 2-D
Practice Using Your Cards

Practice using your cards! This is vital in making lasting changes in your mindset and your behavior. As mentioned, keep the cards in your wallet or purse or other handy place (such as your smartphone) so you can have access to them and **can read them over at least once a day** (we recommend it as one of the first things you do as you start your day). In addition, you'll want the cards nearby so you can turn to them when experiencing an urge to binge eat.

When reading over your Commitment Card, in particular, try to slow yourself down by taking several deep breaths. Try to capture that place deep within you, in your heart of hearts, that is firmly committed to a higher quality of life, that recognizes that using food is costing you more than you can afford to keep paying. Bring to mind how you felt when you wrote your commitment. Try to stay with that feeling, that firm commitment, and the strength and clarity that accompany it.

We realize that depending on how much time it took you to complete the exercises within this chapter, you may not have many days before moving on to the next chapter (if you are aiming to finish one chapter a week). That's OK! The point now is to make your cards so you'll have them available for the rest of this program and beyond.

❑ I have put my cards where I can always get to them easily.

❑ I have read over my cards at least once a day.

We also want to say one more time:

CONGRATULATIONS ON MAKING THE COMMITMENT!

3

Discussing Program Goals
and the Tools to Get You There

The overall goal of this program is to get you the life you want, including stopping binge eating and other related problem behaviors. However, we know that when you have a complex long-term goal, it's often helpful to break it down into smaller steps. This chapter is a great example of that. We have a lot of information we want to share with you that we've broken into three smaller pieces. It's still going to be a long chapter, though, and we congratulate you in advance for sticking with it! The first piece discusses the program's goals. The second introduces you to the Diary Card. We've saved the best for the last piece, in which we introduce you to mindfulness skills.

Program Goals

Getting the life you want has been broken down into the four steps described below. It's important to tackle these steps in sequence, as each relies on achieving the preceding ones.

The Steps to Get the Life You Want

Step 1: Stop any behaviors that interfere with using this program.

Step 2: Stop binge eating.

Step 3: Decrease other eating-related problem behaviors.

Step 4: Decrease other (noneating) problem behaviors.

Step 1: Stop Any Behaviors That Interfere with Using This Program

The reason that stopping *any* behaviors that interfere with using this program is so crucial is that if you could have stopped binge eating on your own, you would not be using this book. If this program is to work for you, you have to be actively engaged—reading the chapters, completing the assigned exercises and homework, and learning how to apply the skills. This will help you keep the commitment you made in Chapter 2—to turn to this program before turning to food. Any behavior that gets in the way of your being actively engaged must be a top priority. Let's say one of our patients is arriving late for her therapy sessions. This means she ends up missing much of the material being taught. Although that patient's goal is to stop binge eating, the first step in treatment is to address why she is missing sessions and what we can do to have her come on time. For example, she may have a relational issue with her therapist that's causing her to be continually late. Or perhaps her partner is critical of her participation in the program and they argue before she leaves for each session. There could be any number of reasons. And whatever the reason, our first goal is to identify the obstacle and resolve it. Your active participation and commitment to this program are essential for your success, so your top priority is making sure you take care of anything that gets in the way of your involvement.

Step 2: Stop Binge Eating (Both Large and Small Binges)

The next step to getting the life you want is to stop binge eating. While a binge is usually defined as experiencing a loss of control while ingesting a large or excessive amount of food (for example, the equivalent of two full meals or three main courses, such as three full servings of lasagna), research shows that the sense of loss of control may be more important than the amount of food eaten. For this reason, if you feel out of control while eating an amount that most people *wouldn't* consider excessive (e.g., two standard-sized cookies), in this program you'll count that as a binge but record it as a small one. Both kinds of binges are types of emotional eating, and it is important to stop all binge eating to live up to your fullest potential. If you have both large and small binges, though, we recommend working on stopping your large binges first.

Step 3: Decrease Other Eating-Related Problem Behaviors

The next step to getting the life you want is to decrease/stop other eating-related problem behaviors. We include here any eating-related problem behaviors that are not considered binges. As we've said, we don't want you to get too caught up in definitions or labels, but we've found it helpful to separate binge eating, or eating with a sense of loss of control (Step 2), from other eating-related problem behaviors:

- **Emotional eating** is eating primarily to relieve emotional discomfort rather than physical hunger. It includes binge eating as well as eating that doesn't involve a loss of control. Emotional eating is problematic whether or not you feel a loss of control, because when you eat in response to intense emotions you are strengthening the connection between emotional discomfort and eating. In addition, by avoiding the opportunity to learn and practice adaptive ways to cope with your emotions, you will be more likely to engage in emotional eating or escalate to binge eating when you're faced with triggers.

- **Mindless eating** is eating without paying attention or without awareness. Some of our patients say that once they realize how much they've already eaten, they end up binge eating in frustration on whatever food remains or seek out even more (John does this, which you'll read more about in Chapter 8).

- **Impulsively breaking a balanced food plan** (if you have one) can overlap with emotional eating, but we focus on it separately because some of our patients who try to follow balanced food plans have run into difficulty because of unplanned snacking, eating larger portions than they'd planned, and so forth. Their emotional response to having had unplanned food, such as feeling guilty or ashamed, often sets them up for a full-fledged binge. We saw this in Chapter 1 with Leticia, who decided that because she had already "blown it," she might as well move straight into a binge and begin her plan again the next day. This decision to give up and surrender to food is called *capitulating*. Capitulating may seem passive, but it is actually an active decision to shut down and close off your options not to binge eat. The truth is that you always have a choice to binge or not, even if it doesn't seem like it.

This assumes, however, that your food plan is not an overly restrictive one that leaves you too physically hungry and therefore more vulnerable to bingeing. We discuss overly restrictive food plans in more detail in Chapter 10. As we mentioned in the Introduction, we recommend reading this section (on pages 176–178) now before proceeding if you are attempting to lose or keep off weight.

Undereating sets you up physiologically to be more vulnerable to binge eating because physical hunger is very uncomfortable and very difficult to tolerate.

- **Urges to binge** as well as **cravings and preoccupation with food** are other eating-related problem behaviors. You may have noticed that many people who binge eat tend to think about food a great deal. We view continuously thinking about food as a problem eating behavior because it distracts you from distressing emotions in ineffective ways that can lead to binge eating.

 • **Apparently irrelevant behaviors (AIBs)** occur when you tell yourself that your behavior is not relevant to binge eating, but you know deep down that it is. Examples of AIBs might be buying a tempting dessert "for company" when you know your preoccupation with that dessert will likely lead to a binge. Another common AIB is not weighing yourself, which deprives you of important feedback about the consequences of your eating. By interfering with awareness, not weighing yourself permits you to pretend that your binge-eating behaviors don't really matter that much. AIBs are often unconscious but will become more apparent as you use the program.

Step 4: Decrease Other (Noneating) Problem Behaviors

Once you have taken the first three steps, you're ready to stop other problem behaviors. As we mentioned in the Introduction, these can include overspending, overexercising, and/or overworking—see the box on page 66. Any behavior you engage in to avoid, or numb, or escape emotional discomfort (including avoiding social activities) can ultimately increase your vulnerability to binge eat. Engaging in these problem behaviors reinforces the unhealthy connection between feeling emotional distress and turning to unhealthy behaviors that are not in line with your core values. Fortunately, the skills we teach apply to both noneating and eating-related problem behaviors.

 Consider these steps to be long-term goals to help you be free of binge eating and remain so. The program will help you learn many skills that you can apply to your own behavior patterns or habits so you can achieve your goals.

Keeping Track of Progress: The Diary Card

The key to making changes and learning new behaviors is to practice. This applies to all kinds of learning—playing music, practicing a sport, learning a foreign language, and so forth. It especially applies to learning to change a long-standing behavior such as binge eating.

 To help you keep track of the changes you make during this program, you will be filling out a Diary Card each day of every week. This Diary Card will also be a place to chart your practice of newly acquired skills, as well as to record your experience of different emotions (e.g., anger, sadness, fear, happiness). The purpose of the Diary Card is to help you notice connections between your emotions and your urges or actual use of problem eating behaviors.

Examples of Noneating Problem Behaviors

Do any of the following descriptions sound familiar to you?

Jessica: Overspending. "I notice that especially when I'm sticking to my food plan, or when I have had a difficult day with my kids, I spend a lot more money. It seems that whenever I'm feeling down or antsy or someone hurts my feelings I want to log on to Amazon or go to the mall. There's something about buying things that just makes me feel better. I buy things I don't really need and definitely spend money I shouldn't. But in those moments I feel like I'm in this other zone."

Mariko: Overexercising. "I used to be a marathon runner and am still obsessed with exercise. I usually fit my workout into my schedule; if not, I feel completely stressed out. I even exercise when I'm injured because otherwise I start to feel guilty, like I'll become lazy and my weight will get out of control. I skip other things so that I can exercise, even avoiding events that are important to me like my daughter's dance recital. Sometimes I worry I'm using exercise as a way to escape my life—escape having to think or feel."

Kelsey: Overworking. "I have always worked fast-paced and demanding jobs in high tech. My work is never 'done'—there's always something else to check on or to finish. My family complains that I don't seem to really be with them even when we're together at home. And it's true, I never seem to be able to fully turn off. I'm always in work mode, almost always anxious and moving on to address the next crisis. I'm not even quite sure who I'd be if I didn't have so much to do. When I try to engage in activities not related to my job, there's always a part of me thinking about what I 'should' be doing for work."

Another important function of the Diary Card is to give you a chance to describe your feelings about the program. Changing your behaviors around food is usually extremely challenging. In fact, it is likely one of the hardest goals, if not the very hardest, you will ever attempt to achieve. As mentioned, Step 1 is to identify and stop behaviors that interfere with making use of this program. For this reason, the Diary Card asks you to rate the urge to quit this program or to engage in other behaviors that interfere with your full participation such as not reading the chapters, not completing the assigned exercises and homework, or not practicing how to apply the skills. If you notice you are giving yourself high ratings regarding urges to quit or to not participate *fully*, it would be a good time to go back to Chapter 2 to review the reasons that you committed to stop binge eating. In addition, if you're working through this program with a therapist (or other trusted, supportive person), this would most likely be the first item on your agenda to address.

As part of this program, you may wish to obtain a weekly measure of your weight and record it on the Diary Card. Regardless of how often you are weighing yourself now, for the duration of this program, we recommend weighing yourself no more than once a week. We have found that patients who weigh themselves more than once a week tend to focus on the fluctuations, which are not meaningful. This can trigger guilt, shame, and other emotions that make you vulnerable to binge eating. On the other hand, not weighing yourself at all allows you to avoid reality. What we're suggesting is a middle path where you can use the information to think about your longer-term goals but not set yourself up for failure. To make it easier to keep to this recommendation, it often helps to pick a specific day and time to weigh yourself.

You can refer to the Diary Card on pages 70–71 as you read through the instructions in the box on pages 68–69. (See the box at the end of the table of contents for information on printing out blank Diary Cards.) The skills on the second page of the Diary Card are listed in the order they are taught in this program. (If you want to make each card a single sheet of paper, you can make double-sided photocopies or print on both sides of your paper.)

EXERCISE 1 Start to Use Your Diary Card Today

Start today with filling out the Diary Card! To help you remember to fill it out every day, tie filling out your Diary Card to a specific event or ritual that is part of your end-of-day routine. Some people keep their Diary Cards on their nightstand, where they'll see them right when they get into bed and can fill them out before going to sleep.

a. **Take a moment and make a plan** for when you will fill out your Diary Card. Write it below.

   My plan for how I will fill out my Diary Card daily (ideally right before going to sleep) is:

   _____

   _____

b. **Begin practicing the first skill listed on your Diary Card, Renewing My Commitment (Pros/Cons).**

   • One way to practice is to begin your day by reading over the pros/cons on the card you created in Homework Exercise 2-A. Then say, either out

Instructions for Completing Your Diary Card

Completing your Diary Card is an essential component of this program. A few tips for using the Diary Cards:

Try not to judge the information you record on your Diary Card as being "bad" or "good." (Adopting a nonjudgmental stance is a tool we will discuss in much more detail later.)

- Complete the Diary Card every day so you don't forget details important to your success.

- Make filling out the card one of the last things you do before going to sleep so you don't "forget" to record a binge episode, for example, that occurred after you filled out the card earlier in the day.

Completing the Front of the Diary Card

Use one Diary Card for each week. Start by filling out the dates of the week. Record your weight and the day on which you weighed yourself. At the end of the week, check off how frequently you filled out the card. Also, rate on a scale of 0–6 the strongest urge you experienced throughout the past week to quit the program or engage in other behaviors that interfere with actively getting the most out of the program. (Keep in mind that it's OK to *want* to quit or *want* to read through the exercises instead of actively trying them; it doesn't mean you have to act on these urges!)

For each day:

- Record the number (if any) of large or small binge episodes.

- Circle "Y" or "N" to indicate whether you had any other problem behaviors that day. Do the same for AIBs. If you did, describe the other problem behaviors or AIBs in the space provided on the Diary Card.

- To help you notice patterns in the connections between your emotional experiences and your problem behaviors, the Diary Card asks you to track the emotions you experienced each day. We listed common emotions, based on our experience with our patients, and left a column for you to fill in with ones that we left out. Refer to the legend and choose the number from the scale (0–6) that best represents your highest rating for the day. The key characteristics to consider when making your rating are intensity (strength of the emotion) and duration (how long it lasted).

Completing the Skills Section of the Diary Card

Go down the column listing all of the skills and circle the days you used each skill. If there are days you did not practice or use any of the skills, then circle those days opposite the last line, which states, "Did not practice/use any skills." Also, make sure to check off how frequently you filled out the skills section of the Diary Card during the week. This helps make clear whether you were checking in with yourself each day or perhaps filled out the card once or twice, basing your practice of the skills on your memory for the past week or so.

Be sure to save your completed Diary Cards. You'll be referring to them at various points in the program (e.g., in Chapter 7 and Chapter 13), and we'll offer you specific suggestions based on your review of your progress. If you're working with a therapist or other guide, you'll want to share your Diary Cards with him or her to review your weekly progress.

---

loud or silently: "Today I am renewing my commitment to stop binge eating and to turn to this program first before turning to food."

- Choose your own most effective way to practice (and feel free to change it over time). Some other ideas patients have come up with include reading over their Commitment Card (created in Homework Exercise 2-B) or Motivation Card (created in Homework Exercise 2-C), programming their phone so that an automatic message with their commitment on it is sent every day during a time they tend to be vulnerable (e.g., every afternoon at 3:00 P.M.), reading short passages from books that inspire them, and looking at inspirational pictures that remind them of the future they want for themselves.

My plan for practicing my first skill, Renewing My Commitment (Pros/Cons), is to:

_____

_____

_____

Introducing Mindfulness Skills

We mentioned in the Introduction that we will be teaching you three categories of skills that build on one another. The first of these is *mindfulness*, which forms the bedrock for learning the skills taught in the later modules; *emotion regulation*; and *distress tolerance*. The practice of mindfulness can be traced back at least 3,000

Diary Card (page 1 of 2)

Week beginning ____/____/____ ending ____/____/____

This week I filled out this section: ☐ Daily ☐ 4–6× ☐ 2–3× ☐ Once

Highest urge over past week to quit program/engage in program-interfering behaviors (0–6)*: _____

Date I weighed myself: ____/____/____   Weight: _____

Eating and Other Behaviors

Day	Urge to binge*	Binge episodes — Number of large episodes	Binge episodes — Number of small episodes	Any other eating and non-eating-related problem behaviors**?	Any AIBs**? (apparently irrelevant behaviors)	Anger (0–6)	Sadness (0–6)	Fear/ anxiety/ restless-ness (0–6)	Shame (0–6)	Embarrass-ment (0–6)	Guilt (0–6)	Boredom/ loneliness (0–6)	Pride (0–6)	Happiness (0–6)	Content-ment (0–6)	Other (fill in) ___ ___ (0–6)
												Emotion				
Mon				Y N	Y N											
Tue				Y N	Y N											
Wed				Y N	Y N											
Thu				Y N	Y N											
Fri				Y N	Y N											
Sat				Y N	Y N											
Sun				Y N	Y N											

*Rate from 0 to 6 the highest rating for the day or week (0 = did not experience it—the urge, thought, or feeling—to 6 = experienced it intensely).

**Describe other problem behaviors and AIBs: _____

_____

_____

From *The DBT® Solution for Emotional Eating* by Debra L. Safer, Sarah Adler, and Philip C. Masson. Copyright © 2018 The Guilford Press. Purchasers of this book can photocopy and/or download an enlarged version of this form (see the box at the end of the table of contents).

Instructions: Circle the days you used each skill.   This week I filled out this section: ☐ Daily   ☐ 4–6×   ☐ 2–3×   ☐ Once

	Day						
Renewing my commitment (pros/cons)	Mon	Tue	Wed	Thu	Fri	Sat	Sun
Wise mind	Mon	Tue	Wed	Thu	Fri	Sat	Sun
Diaphragmatic breathing	Mon	Tue	Wed	Thu	Fri	Sat	Sun
Dialectical thinking	Mon	Tue	Wed	Thu	Fri	Sat	Sun
Observing: Just noticing	Mon	Tue	Wed	Thu	Fri	Sat	Sun
Adopting a nonjudgmental stance	Mon	Tue	Wed	Thu	Fri	Sat	Sun
Focusing on one thing in the moment	Mon	Tue	Wed	Thu	Fri	Sat	Sun
Being effective	Mon	Tue	Wed	Thu	Fri	Sat	Sun
Mindful eating	Mon	Tue	Wed	Thu	Fri	Sat	Sun
Urge surfing	Mon	Tue	Wed	Thu	Fri	Sat	Sun
Mindfulness of my current emotion	Mon	Tue	Wed	Thu	Fri	Sat	Sun
Radically accepting my current emotion	Mon	Tue	Wed	Thu	Fri	Sat	Sun
Decreasing vulnerability/building mastery	Mon	Tue	Wed	Thu	Fri	Sat	Sun
Building positive experiences (avoiding avoiding)	Mon	Tue	Wed	Thu	Fri	Sat	Sun
Being mindful of positive emotions	Mon	Tue	Wed	Thu	Fri	Sat	Sun
Half-smiling	Mon	Tue	Wed	Thu	Fri	Sat	Sun
Crisis survival skills	Mon	Tue	Wed	Thu	Fri	Sat	Sun
Coping ahead	Mon	Tue	Wed	Thu	Fri	Sat	Sun
Did not practice/use any skills	Mon	Tue	Wed	Thu	Fri	Sat	Sun

years, with famous practitioners including the Buddha. Mindfulness has been a core element of many Eastern philosophies as well as religious and spiritual practices. More recently, mindfulness has been studied scientifically in the West and has demonstrated a positive effect on managing emotional distress.

In its broadest sense, mindfulness is simply keeping something in mind, being aware, and/or noticing what is happening. Mindfulness skills teach you to be involved in the present moment without judging the situation or yourself. Some patients worry that mindfulness is an abstract concept that they cannot possibly learn or practice. But mindfulness means simply paying attention in a particular way. It is a skill everyone can develop. Many who have practiced mindfulness attest that it significantly enhances the pleasure and eases the pain they experience in their lives.

We saw in Chapter 1 how Angela felt compelled to binge because food offered her a temporary escape from distressing emotions. Mindfulness skills helped Angela by teaching her to take a step back from these triggering situations so that she was less emotionally reactive and could use her skills to prevent a binge. They will help you too. Mindfulness skills empower you to notice automatic links between your emotions and binge eating. For example, mindfulness increases your ability to be aware that feeling discouraged leads you to experience urges to binge eat. Additionally, mindfulness empowers you to use this awareness to decide what other skills you may wish to use to manage your feelings.

The basic skills of mindfulness are simple but require practice over time. It's no different from learning any other skill. For example, the mechanics of lifting weights can be grasped rather quickly, but regular practice at the gym is required for you to build muscle. And if you stop practicing, those mindfulness "muscles," just like physical muscles, weaken.

Mindfulness is also a type of meditation, as discussed in the box on page 73.

The Three States of Mind

Mindfulness proposes that there are three major states of mind: reasonable mind, emotion mind, and wise mind. Each of these states of mind influences your behavior.

REASONABLE MIND

Reasonable mind is a state of mind in which your behaviors are controlled primarily by rational thinking and logic. They are based on the facts. Examples of situations in which reasonable mind predominates include balancing your checkbook, solving a logic or math problem, following a map, or planning and evaluating a course of action. Your mindset in reasonable mind could be described as "cool."

Mindfulness as Meditation

Practicing the mindfulness skills the way we teach them to you in this program does not require a meditation practice. Skills practice will be sufficient for obtaining full benefit in helping you stop binge eating. Some of our patients wish to develop their mindfulness skills further through a meditation practice (and some have had past experience with other types of meditation). There are many avenues to pursue to learn more about mindfulness meditation. Apps we particularly like include Headspace (*www.headspace.com*), which offers simple 10-minute guided meditations, and InsightTimer (*https://insighttimer.com*), which is free.

Being in reasonable mind can be very beneficial. But if you are using only reason and logic to determine your actions, you may overlook important aspects of a situation. For example, reasonable mind might tell you: "There's nothing more to losing weight than burning more calories than I eat. It should be as simple as that." Ignoring the influence of your emotions on your eating behavior and operating solely from your reasonable mind can set you up to feel like a failure and cause you to give up.

EMOTION MIND

The other end of the continuum is emotion mind—the mindset in which your behavior is controlled primarily by your current emotional state. In emotion mind, your thinking is "hot." Rational decisions are very difficult and facts are often distorted or intensified to match your mood. It's as if you are strapped to a runaway horse and have no reins to guide its direction or slow it down. When "emotion

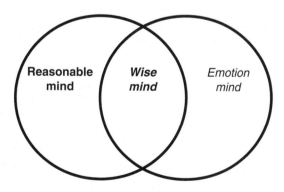

The three states of mind.

mind" takes over, it can feel like a flood of energy or a wash of depression over which you have no influence or control.

This is not to say that emotions are in any way "bad." Information from our emotional responses is essential for living a rich life and can be a powerful motivator. Emotions are "hard-wired" and necessary for survival. Misery and distress can motivate us to change. Intense love can compel a parent to run through a fire to save a child. But acting based solely on your emotions can also lead to out-of-control behaviors that are out of touch with your core values.

EXERCISE 2   When Your Emotions Are in Control

a. Can you think of a time when your **emotions were in control** and led to **behaviors that were helpful to you?** Write your response below.

_____

_____

_____

_____

_____

_____

Kat wrote the following:

My decision to leave my last job and take a job my friend offered me with her company involved my emotions being in control. I felt like I was slowly dying, putting in long hours doing work that didn't interest me. The thing was that the money was good and my friend's company, at the time, was a little unstable. The reasonable part of my mind told me to concentrate on the good pay and ignore the rest. But once I had this other opportunity my emotion mind kicked in. I was able to really feel how much I hated the old job and to recognize on an emotional level that no amount of financial compensation was worth it. So, I immediately gave notice. Having my emotions in control was helpful or I'd probably just have stuck it out and remained miserable. Things have turned out really well at my friend's company. Now I have more time and energy to devote to what I really care about—singing—and the drop in income hasn't been difficult to adjust to at all.

b. Can you think of a time when your **emotions were in control** and led you to **behaviors you regretted?** Write your response below.

_____

_____

_____

_____

_____

Kat wrote:

Every binge feels like that! The worst one I had recently was the one with the chocolate truffles. I was feeling so awful and completely couldn't stand looking in the mirror. It just activated all my insecurities about aging and what led Tom to have an affair last year.

WISE MIND

Wise mind is the state of mind that synthesizes both reasonable and emotion mind. What we mean is that when you are accessing wise mind, you include information from reasonable mind's logical thinking and emotion mind's focus on feelings. But wise mind is more than the sum of its parts. Wise mind taps into your intuition, inner wisdom, and experience of truth. You are in wise mind when your best self takes over—when you're aware of both your emotions and your logical thinking but are not controlled by either. Your wise mind is the part of you that gives yourself your very best advice (whether or not you always listen!). Wise mind combines your logical thinking (reasonable mind) with how you feel (emotion mind) so that you can make decisions from a deep and centered part of yourself where you're in touch with your values. Other terms for your wise mind include your true self, your spirit, your heart of hearts, and your consciousness.

People experience being in wise mind differently—there isn't a single, universal way. Many, however, recognize being in wise mind when their decisions come from a very core place. There's a sense of knowing something in a very deep, integrated way. The box on page 76 gives some examples of questions we've been asked about what wise mind would or wouldn't say.

Sometimes your wise mind's advice or response may be not to act at all, but to maintain awareness of your urge to act. An example would involve being aware of your urges to binge but not acting on these urges because your wise mind knows doing so would be self-destructive.

Would Wise Mind Say This?

Question: Would wise mind give me permission to binge?

Response: Before wise mind would do anything, it would notice your urges and, without judgment, become aware of all aspects of your experience. We have never seen wise mind suggest acting mindlessly in ways that go against your firmly held values—and bingeing is, by definition, mindless.

Question: Would wise mind tell me it's OK to stop practicing the skills if they take up too much time?

Response: Wise mind would validate that the skills *do* take time and remind you, without any judgment, that if you're finding time to binge you can find time to practice the skills.

Question: Should I expect my wise mind's advice to feel peaceful and calm?

Response: Not necessarily! Sometimes your wise mind may have to jump up and down and wave its arms to get your attention so you change your behavior. While you may find a certain peace in acknowledging the soundness of wise mind's advice, your decision to follow your wise mind may feel quite difficult and uncomfortable.

You may wonder, like some of our patients do, whether or not you even have a wise mind! Please see the box on the facing page.

The following experiential exercise will help you increase access to your wise mind.

EXERCISE 3 Finding Your Wise Mind Practice

"Start by sitting comfortably in a chair. Find a place for your eyes to focus gently so that you're not distracted. Let the chair fully support you—your feet on the floor and your hands on your knees or lap. Imagine that a string is running through your head up to the ceiling keeping you upright. If you find your mind wandering, notice this and bring it gently back to the exercise.

"Begin by following your breath. This is often a helpful way to facilitate awareness as it anchors you to the present moment. You don't have to do any type of special breathing, just be aware of your breath. It may help to initially note the sensation of air moving in and out of your nostrils. As you breathe, try to go 'into yourself' and find a place of calmness, of peace. Some people find it helpful to imagine themselves as a stone or pebble slowly sinking into a warm lake. The surface of the lake has ripples, but as you sink down deeper, the water becomes still. Imagine yourself floating down . . . gently . . . slowly. Allow yourself to sink and settle calmly into the sandy bottom of the lake. You are at rest. The sandy bottom is fully supporting you.

"From this quiet, peaceful place, you have distance from the choppy surface and you can get in touch with your core values. Operating from your wise mind, you can see and respond to what is—to reality. You are your true self, your spirit, your consciousness. You are open to experience itself. Let your deep inner wisdom guide your actions so that they're consistent with your values. What does your wise mind think about stopping binge eating? How would your wise mind advise you to approach this program? Take time to feel what it is like to have access to this part of yourself, to this inner conviction and wisdom. When you are ready, take three deep, slow, flowing breaths and leave this image."

What If I Don't Have a Wise Mind?

Everyone has a wise mind, whether or not you believe this. Possessing a wise mind is like possessing a heart—it is part of the definition of what it means to be human. One reason you might wonder if you have a wise mind is that binge eating and other problematic eating behaviors interfere with being in touch with your wise mind—with your best self, your clarity of being, that inner sense of what's important. So you may not have had full access to your wise mind. Or perhaps you find it hard at times to figure out the difference between what your wise mind advises versus "guidance" from your emotion mind or reasonable mind. For instance, would wise mind tell you to finish the entire container of ice cream because, with none left, you won't have to deal with it the next day? Or would wise mind suggest eating as little as possible the day before a party as a useful strategy to save calories for later? If you're not sure, sometimes it can be easier to figure out if the advice is coming from your wise mind by picturing talking to a loved one who is struggling. Imagine the other person explaining why it's a good idea for her to finish the ice cream or skip the meals. Would you listen and agree that the advice is in her best interests? We suspect that, deep down, you know you'd never agree that eating until the container was empty or skipping meals was a good strategy for a beloved friend to follow. By thinking of what you'd say to your friend, you're less likely to be thrown off track by emotion mind or reasonable mind's distortions and instead grasp intuitively when you're trying to rationalize acting self-destructively.

With awareness, attention, and lots of practice with the exercises in this chapter and others, you *will* be able to increase your access to your wise mind.

What did you experience? Write about it below.

_____

_____

_____

_____

_____

Kat wrote:

I experienced a sense of calm as I started out. I tried to imagine myself as a pebble sinking down slowly but got a little worried about how I would breathe (even though I knew I was a pebble!). So I tried to just stay with my breathing and sense of calm and tried to ask myself what my wise mind thinks about stopping binge eating and this program. I felt my wise mind was supporting me to stick with this, telling me that I deserved to stop binge eating and live according to my values. My wise mind told me to keep doing what I'm doing.

Patients sometimes ask us what they can do to deepen their access to their wise mind. In addition to practicing the preceding exercise, we recommend they try to think of ways they can create calm moments as these tend to be particularly useful for tapping into wise mind. Some examples patients have used include:

- Taking a walk on a nature trail
- Journaling
- Praying
- Taking deep breaths
- Thinking about what you would advise your child or other loved one to do

We encourage you to try these or come up with your own ideas—be creative! For homework we will ask you to make sure you try out some ways to practice accessing your wise mind over the next week. But, as with all the skills in the program, you should continue to use any that you find helpful both throughout treatment and afterwards.

Diaphragmatic Breathing

This next mindfulness skill, called diaphragmatic breathing, is deceptively simple. Don't be fooled. It is remarkably powerful and can be extremely helpful in breaking the pattern of behaviors that lead to binge eating.

Those of you who have practiced meditation or yoga may have already been introduced to diaphragmatic breathing. This is an opportunity to reinforce its use.

What happens physically when you experience very strong emotions? For many people, the rate of breathing changes, the heart rate speeds up, and the body starts to sweat or feel clammy. Some people feel dizzy and/or notice an uncomfortable clenching in their gut. These physical sensations can increase the original feelings of distress and cause you to turn to food for relief.

Diaphragmatic breathing, or deep breathing, interrupts the physiological and emotional manifestations of distress. It can also facilitate mindfulness, which involves focusing your attention and increasing your awareness of the present moment. One way to practice mindfulness is to notice your breath as it flows in and out, anchoring you in the "here and now" of the current moment.

Learning and practicing deep breathing and focusing on your breath can help you stop preoccupations with food. When you feel an urge to binge eat, you can calm yourself and ride out the urge. Deep breathing is very helpful for relieving emotional distress and physical tensions that have built up and that can trigger the urge to binge. You're replacing the eating behavior and focus on food with deep breathing and a focus on your breathing. Your breath is always with you, so the skill of deep breathing is readily available, always right under your nose.

EXERCISE 4 Diaphragmatic Breathing Practice

Just a note: Some of our patients are initially uncomfortable with this exercise because it involves paying attention to their abdomens or stomach area—a part of the body many judge harshly. It can feel especially triggering to focus on having the abdomen expand. Others find that simply paying attention to their breathing initially makes them more anxious. A useful strategy that can help in either case is to practice diaphragmatic breathing while doing something else at the same time, such as taking a slow walk. But keep in mind that by the end of this program, when we ask patients to rate the skill they found most useful, diaphragmatic breathing is often at the top of the list! We encourage you to stick with the skill because of how effectively deep breathing interrupts the physiological and emotional manifestations of distress and anxiety.

"Practice taking slow, regular, flowing breaths associated with expanding your abdomen, as opposed to shallow breaths from your upper chest or throat. It might be helpful to imagine a balloon inside your abdomen that is slowly filling up with air, then slowly deflating, then slowly inflating, and so on.

"The rate of breathing should be about 10–12 breaths per minute. This means taking about 3 seconds to slowly inhale and about 3 seconds to slowly exhale. Inhale and exhale through your nose. As you inhale, slowly count ONE, TWO, THREE. As you exhale, silently say to yourself "relax" or "calm." Do this up to a count of 10 and then start again at one. Try to keep your awareness on your slow breathing.

"If you wish, place a hand on your abdomen so you can feel it slowly move in and out. Try to keep your awareness on your breath, letting it flow. Your mind will wander, but the more you practice, the easier it will be to bring your attention back to your breathing. Be patient. Try not to judge yourself. Don't worry about having to do anything fancy!"

Write about your practice of diaphragmatic breathing below. What did you notice? Did your rate of breathing slow? Did you experience any change in your anxiety level? How hard or difficult was it to stay present with your breathing? When your mind wandered, how long did it take before you noticed?

_____

_____

_____

_____

Kat wrote:

I used to do yoga, so I'm familiar with this type of belly breathing. I noticed that as I breathed in and out I felt calmer and less anxious. I thought counting was helpful. I was able to stay present with my breathing for about 5 breaths before my mind wandered.

You can use this skill when you have worries, anxiety, or anytime you notice your emotions becoming more intense. Simply slow down and focus on your breathing. In addition to practicing this skill when you are feeling intense emotions, practice it regularly no matter what is going on. The more you practice diaphragmatic breathing, the more aware you'll be of how your breathing pattern can serve to anchor and calm your mind.

Chapter 3 Summary

In this chapter we reviewed the goals of this program and the steps to help you achieve them. The most crucial of these steps is to stop any behaviors that interfere with using the program. This will enable you to address the all-important goal of stopping binge eating. You'll then have the resources to stop other problem behaviors, first focusing on those that are eating related and then on those that are not eating related.

We then introduced you to an important tool called the Diary Card. Filling out the Diary Card is a way to monitor your progress every day. As you continue to use the Diary Card you can begin to look back and start to spot relationships between your emotions and binge eating. The Diary Card also helps you stay on track!

Finally, we introduced mindfulness, followed by two particular mindfulness skills that many of our patients have identified as being the most useful skills they've learned to reduce urges to binge eat. The first, wise mind, involves integrating information from both reasonable mind and emotion mind to make use of and integrate all ways of knowing. The second skill, diaphragmatic breathing, focuses on having you slow down your rate of respiration. When people experience strong emotions, their breathing often becomes shallow and their heart rate speeds up. Deep breathing dials down physiological and emotional intensity. It is deceptively simple. Practicing it when you are already calm can help keep you calm, and using it when you are becoming upset can help you restore equanimity.

Homework

Remember to check the box after you have completed each homework assignment.

HOMEWORK EXERCISE 3-A
Fill Out Your Diary Card Each Day

Throughout the rest of this program you should fill out the Diary Card once a day. Ideally, keep it with you during the day to help you maintain accurate records of skills you've practiced and your use of the targeted behaviors. It is helpful to review the card at the end of the day to make sure that all the skills practiced and all targeted behaviors were recorded. Remember to keep all your Diary Cards!

❑ I have filled out my Diary Card daily this week.

HOMEWORK EXERCISE 3-B
Accessing and Using Your Wise Mind

Over the next week, make sure to practice *accessing* your wise mind in Exercise 3 (Finding Your Wise Mind Practice) at least once more. In addition, practice *using* your wise mind at least once a day for the next week by asking yourself, "What would my wise mind say?" and following your wise mind's suggestions. For example, practice asking this question before even making everyday decisions such as whether to add an extra errand to your to-do list, go to sleep earlier, turn down an invitation, or let someone else "win."

❑ I have practiced accessing my wise mind using Exercise 3 at least once.

❑ I have practiced using my wise mind at least once a day, asking myself, "What would my wise mind say?" and then following its suggestions.

HOMEWORK EXERCISE 3-C

Maintaining Connection with Your Wise Mind

Having accessed your wise mind, what do you think could help you maintain a connection to this part of yourself throughout this program and the challenges you will face? Write your thoughts below.

_____

_____

_____

_____

_____

_____

_____

Kat wrote:

I think one of the best ways to maintain my connection to my wise mind is to make it a daily habit. Otherwise I can get caught up in my life and forget—especially at the times I need this connection most, like if I were to get off track. Checking in with my wise mind in the morning when I'm brushing my teeth and then again at night would help to make it a habit.

HOMEWORK EXERCISE 3-D

Practicing Diaphragmatic Breathing Twice a Day

Practice diaphragmatic breathing twice a day for 1–5 minutes at a time and circle your use of the skill on your Diary Card. Ideally, practice when you are calm. In addition, practice at points throughout your day—for example, when you are driving or taking a walk, when you are on the phone, at work, or at a party. The more you practice, the more likely it is that you will remember to turn to this effective skill if you notice any urges to binge eat.

Write about your experience practicing this skill.

_____

_____

_____

_____

_____

_____

_____

Kat wrote:

This has worked well for me this week. I have been practicing diaphragmatic breathing when I walk to and from the bus stop to work and home. It has been very calming and centering. I found as the week went on that I started using it at other times during the day, like when I was standing in line at the grocery store and when I was on hold on the phone. The more often I use it, the easier it is for me to remember to use it. It also seems to act more quickly—like my body is developing a muscle memory for it.

❑ I have practiced diaphragmatic breathing twice a day this week.

❑ I have read over my cards at least once a day.

4

Learning to Become Your Own
DBT Coach

At this point you should have a clearer picture of how difficulties with managing emotions can keep you trapped in binge eating. You also have learned several skills (renewing your commitment, wise mind, and diaphragmatic breathing) to help you begin to cope more effectively with unpleasant emotional states that may trigger attempts to self-soothe with food.

The next step is to learn to apply those skills in the moment when you find yourself experiencing such intense emotions. To do that, you have to be able to recognize the specific patterns that lead you to binge eat. The more you understand the factors that contribute to your disordered eating, the more likely you are to find ways to change those patterns and prevent them from recurring.

To accomplish this task, we offer the behavioral chain analysis, a tool that enables you to identify exactly what the problem behavior is (the details of where and when you binged), what triggered the binge, the binge's function, and what solutions are available to solve the problem more effectively. Perhaps most important, it gives you a way to sort through and analyze information describing your eating behaviors without letting your emotions, negative thoughts, or judgments interfere with your objectivity.

Using the behavioral chain analysis, you can become your own DBT coach. Taking on this role not only allows you to stop binge eating while you're actively working through this program but also enables you to maintain this progress afterward. Even if you have slips in the future, you know what to do to get yourself quickly back on track.

How the Behavioral Chain Analysis Works

When binge eating is an overlearned behavior, as it is for many of our patients, it seems to start before you know what's happening. Do you sometimes feel you can't really describe how you got from point A, where you were not binge eating, to point B, where you were? This is part of that "out of control" feeling that many binge eaters experience. "It's almost as if the binge happens *to* me," they say. "There's a blurry quality. I know I'm the one doing everything, but I don't feel aware of all of it."

The behavioral chain analysis helps you see that you're not catapulted into a binge by some uncontrollable outside force but that the process of getting from point A to point B is made up of a sequence of discernable events. These are the links in the behavioral chain, as shown in the diagram below. When you can identify each one, you gain the power to break the chain. You don't have to end up at the problem behavior shown in the diagram.

By analyzing the events both leading up to and following your binge, you will be able to prevent future binge episodes and eventually stop problematic behaviors already in progress. Breaking any one of the links on the chain of behaviors that lead to binge eating will cause the whole chain of behaviors to fall apart. Let's take a closer look at the chain.

• **Vulnerability factors:** Factors like illness and fatigue can make you particularly susceptible to the chain of events that lead to a binge episode. They weaken your resilience and make you more vulnerable to the difficult emotions raised by a prompting event.

• **Prompting event:** This link represents what triggered the chain of events toward the binge. It could be anything from having an argument with your partner to looking in the mirror to seeing a favorite food.

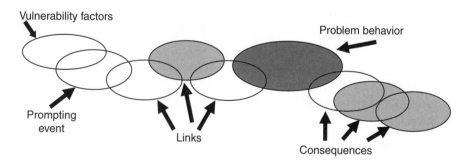

The components of a behavioral chain.

• **Links:** These are the specific actions, feelings, thoughts, and other experiences that explain what took place between being triggered by the prompting event and engaging in the problem behavior. Leticia's bingeing on her mother's home cooking, described in Chapter 1, was prompted by the aromas of food she loved. The links in the behavioral chain that followed included overwhelming desire (emotion) to eat more than the tiny serving she had vowed to have, serving herself much more food than that (action), the recognition that she had broken her diet (thought), which made her feel ashamed (emotions). The result was a binge.

• **Problem behavior:** In this program, this is typically a binge-eating episode, although it could be another eating-related behavior (e.g., emotional eating, mindless eating, AIB) or a non-eating-related behavior (see Chapter 3). For Leticia, it was a binge that involved eating all the food she had hoped to avoid.

• **Consequences:** These are what occur as a result of a binge episode (or other problem behavior), both immediately afterward and further in the future. For Leticia, the immediate effects of the binge involved slipping into an almost trancelike state in which all she focused on was the sensation of the foods. The longer-term consequences were feeling overly full physically as well as highly self-critical and extremely demoralized.

The immediate consequences provide important information about the function of the binge. The trancelike state allowed Leticia to avoid experiencing her disappointment and other painful emotions related to initially breaking her diet by eating more food than she had planned. She was able to escape into a temporary state where judgment was suspended as she focused entirely on the sensations of the food she was eating. The later consequences, such as Leticia's feelings of utter demoralization, coupled with physical discomfort, may make it more likely for another binge to occur. The feelings of dejection and discomfort may lead her to seek overly simplistic solutions. For example, instead of taking the time to step back to recognize the sequence of events that led to and followed her binge, she may miss the opportunity to learn from what happened and instead simply comfort herself with a promise even she doesn't believe that the next dinner will be different and she will not let herself eat more than she has planned. Or her distressing emotions may lead her to declare that her situation is hopeless, that there is no choice but to realize she is doomed by her biochemistry to a life of binge eating. Eventually either mindset would make a next binge more likely, thus linking this chain to yet another.

Once you understand how the behavioral chain fits together, you can analyze it to find ways to break the chain. Each component of the behavioral chain is included in the Behavioral Chain Analysis Form shown on page 88, which is very easy to use:

1. Fill in a brief description of your problem behavior.

2. Describe the prompting event.

3. Circle the types of vulnerability factors that played a role in making you susceptible to the prompting event and include a brief description.

4. List in the table the specific links that took place after the prompting event, leading up to the problem behavior. Then circle a letter to indicate whether the link was an **A**ction, **B**ody Sensation, **C**ognition, **E**vent, or **F**eeling.

5. Identify skillful behaviors you could have used to substitute for the links, which would have allowed you to break the chain.

6. Describe the immediate and longer-term consequences of the binge.

7. Write down your plan to repair the harm that resulted from your problem behavior.

Binge eating is a learned behavior, and that means it can be *un*learned. With the behavioral chain analysis in hand, you now have a tool for unlearning it. It will take some practice to learn how to use the analysis form and become your own DBT coach, but we know you'll find the effort worthwhile. We can't promise that you'll eliminate setbacks or make them less painful, but the behavioral chain analysis will enable you to learn from your slips in a way that you couldn't do in the past. Learning why these slips occur will liberate you from feeling hopelessly stuck. We've said it before, but it bears repeating: Remember, each setback, as undesirable as it is, gives you another chance to learn and practice. You *will* get it!

Step-by-Step Instructions for Filling Out the Behavioral Chain Analysis Form

To give you a good start, we present step-by-step instructions, walking you through an example from one of Angela's behavioral chain analyses, shown on page 89. You first met Angela in the Introduction and reviewed emotion regulation models for two of her binges in Chapter 1. Angela had felt she understood how her emotions and binges were connected, but she wasn't fully aware of all the factors contributing to her binge eating until she started regularly filling out Behavioral Chain Analysis Forms.

　　1. The first step in filling out a Behavioral Chain Analysis Form is **identifying the problem behavior** that you will focus on. As shown in the example, the

Behavioral Chain Analysis Form

1. **Problem behavior** (include date took place _____):

   _____

2. **Prompting event:** _____

   _____

3. **Vulnerability factors** (circle and describe): physical illness, unbalanced sleep, intense emotional states, stressful environment, other:

   _____

4. Describe specific **links on chain** (and circle if **A**ction,   5. Skillful behaviors
   Body sensation, **C**ognition, **E**vent, or **F**eeling)   to substitute

   _____ ABC-EF _____

   _____ ABC-EF _____

   _____ ABC-EF _____

   _____ ABC-EF _____

   _____ ABC-EF _____

   _____ ABC-EF _____

   _____ ABC-EF _____

   _____ ABC-EF _____

   _____ ABC-EF _____

   Mark the key dysfunctional link with an asterisk (*).

6. **What were the consequences of the behavior?**
   Immediate: _____

   _____

   Longer-term: _____

   _____

7. **Plan to repair harm and do things differently next time:**

   _____

   _____

From *The DBT® Solution for Emotional Eating* by Debra L. Safer, Sarah Adler, and Philip C. Masson. Copyright © 2018 The Guilford Press. Purchasers of this book can photocopy and/or download an enlarged version of this form (see the box at the end of the table of contents).

1. **Problem behavior** (include date took place ___Nov. 29___):
   I had a 1-hour binge on junk food Tuesday evening in my car.

2. **Prompting event:** I got in an argument with my husband about our
   upcoming holiday plans.

3. **Vulnerability factors** (circle and describe): physical illness, (unbalanced sleep,) intense
   emotional states, stressful environment, other:
   I had stayed up too late, as I often do, the night before.

4. Describe specific **links on chain** (and circle if **A**ction, **B**ody sensation, **C**ognition, **E**vent, or **F**eeling)

   5. Skillful behaviors to substitute

Links on chain		Skillful behaviors to substitute
I grabbed my things and got into my car	(A)BC-EF	Diaphragmatic breathing, renew commitment—grab this book!
I wondered if I was being selfish. Should I apologize?	AB(C)EF	Wise mind—Remind myself it's ok to not know, it's complicated
I felt sad about how stressful and complicated the holidays had become	ABC-E(F)	Wise mind (will probably tell me my complicated feelings are valid)
I felt my muscles tighten up, I gripped the steering wheel	A(B)C-EF	Diaphragmatic breathing
I felt overwhelmed, confused, sad, and angry	ABC-(EF)	Ask wise mind—what really matters here? Renew commitment
I thought, "I'll show him! I won't come home for hours. I don't care"	AB(C)EF	Renew commitment to stop binge eating, read my 3x5 card
I thought, "I will feel better if I treat myself to some food," and began thinking about what food I could buy*	AB(C)EF	Ask wise mind to remind me how much I'd regret this tomorrow
I felt desire, excitement, and anticipation*	ABC-(EF)	Renew commitment, 3x5 card, (read book if have it), wise mind, breathe
Pulled into a 7-11 store, bought food, then binged in my car	(A)BC-EF	Renew commitment (read book if have it), diaphragmatic breathing

   Mark the key dysfunctional link with an asterisk (*).

6. **What were the consequences of the behavior?**
   Immediate: _____

   Longer-term: _____

7. **Plan to repair harm and do things differently next time:**
   _____
   _____

problem behavior that Angela identified was a binge-eating episode. She includes helpful details such as the date, how long her binge lasted, what types of food she ate, when it took place, and where she was at the time. Although her binge was actually the last event to take place sequentially on the behavioral chain, it is identified in the first section of the Behavioral Chain Analysis Form. This keeps the problematic behavior in focus from the start.

You'll also notice that Angela is focusing on only one binge. We have found that our patients learn much more by filling out a detailed analysis that examines what led to a single episode than they do by attempting to summarize more than one event. The patterns you need to understand will reveal themselves through your attention to specifics, not generalities—even if you feel, as some of our patients do who binge often, that all their binges are the same.

2. Next, **identify the prompting event.** What happened in your environment that started the chain of events that eventually led to the problem behavior? For Angela, the prompting event was an argument with her husband. Earlier, the two of them had agreed that his mother would stay at a hotel during the holidays. However, her husband told Angela that day he'd spoken to his mother earlier and had asked her, without consulting Angela, to stay at their home. Angela summarized this in section 2 of the Behavioral Chain Analysis Form.

3. This next step asks you to identify **vulnerability factors,** both internal and external, that occurred before the prompting event, making you more susceptible to it. Examples are physical illness, fatigue, unbalanced eating, drug or alcohol use, stressful events in the environment, intense negative or positive emotional states (such as loneliness, excitement, desire), and experiencing painful memories. Section 3 on the form lists some of these factors. Circle those that are relevant or add others. There is space to include additional details. On her Behavioral Chain Analysis Form, Angela circled unbalanced sleep as her chief vulnerability factor and mentioned not getting to bed on time the night before. We discuss vulnerability factors in more detail in Chapter 10.

4. The next step is to **describe the specific links,** or sequence of events, that explain how you got from the prompting event to your problem behavior. Basically, what happened first? And what happened next? Do your best to describe the main links in the sequence in which they occurred, but don't get overly caught up. Just fill out the links with your best guess as to their order.

The first link Angela identified after the prompting event of the argument with her husband was grabbing her things and leaving the house. The next link she recalled was that she questioned whether she was being selfish in wanting her husband to stick to the original plan of having his mother stay in a hotel instead of at their house. Although at the time she wasn't quite aware of it, Angela later remembered, as she was filling out the chain, that she then felt deep sadness that something she had been looking forward to, the holidays, had turned into something stressful and complicated. She then recalled being in the car, sensing her muscles being tight as she gripped the steering wheel.

Also part of this step is circling a letter in the column to the right: **A** for your **A**ctions, or things that you said or did (e.g., "I stopped at a grocery store," "I yelled at my child"); **B** for **B**ody sensations (e.g., "a knot in my stomach," "my heart pounding"); **C** for **C**ognitions, or thoughts (e.g., "I look awful in this," "There's no point in trying"); **E** for the **E**vents that took place (e.g., "My boss asked me to stay late," "Got invited to a potluck"); and **F** for your **F**eelings (e.g., angry, overwhelmed, eager, lonely, scared). Look at Angela's form to see how she identified these links.

5. This next step, Section 5 of the form (right-hand column) is extremely important because it involves **identifying what you could have done differently by substituting a skill to break the chain of events.** Look at each of the links you filled out in Step 4 and decide where you could have used a skill instead. Then, in the space opposite that link, describe the skill or behavior you could have used to handle that link differently.

As Angela filled out her form, she realized that if she'd used diaphragmatic breathing even for just a few minutes after grabbing her things and leaving the house, she would likely have disrupted the chain of problematic behaviors. Breathing deeply and slowly, instead of continuing to act, would have given her the opportunity to stop the escalation of distressing thoughts and feelings that resulted in her binge. She also wrote that renewing her commitment by grabbing this book as she went out the door would have helped.

Angela's example of a complete chain identifies many other places where she felt, in retrospect, she could have substituted a skill. Indeed, the more links you identify in Step 4, the more opportunities there are to substitute a skill in Step 5.

Some people are more aware of their feelings, thoughts, actions, and body sensations than others. Angela was able to notice her tense muscles as she gripped the steering wheel, but if you're not typically highly aware of what's happening in your body before or during a binge, don't worry. As you gain experience thinking in terms of the different categories of links, you will find it easier to provide greater detail in Step 4.

This is important because the next time you experience urges to binge, your ability to pay attention, even minimally, to any tension in your body (e.g., your neck or shoulders) means you can add a link describing this body sensation on your Behavioral Chain Analysis Form afterward. Then, in Step 5, you can identify a skill to substitute, such as diaphragmatic breathing, that could have helped you slow down and relax and might have provided an opportunity to break the chain.

We've seen people gain enough mindfulness to become aware that, in that very moment, they are living a link on their chain. This enables them to mentally recognize Step 4 and substitute a skill as part of Step 5, effectively breaking their chain in real time. This facility will come later, with much practice, but it is something to look forward to. For now, know that it's perfectly understandable to find it difficult to provide specific details about what was going on in your mind or body prior to or during your binges.

6. Here you identify both the immediate and longer-term consequences of the problem behavior. In Angela's case, the immediate consequence of her binge was that she no longer cared about the argument with her husband that had seemed so important earlier. She felt detached and numb. The longer-term consequence, after the detachment wore off, was that she was consumed by the regret and remorse that typically followed her binges. Binge eating ultimately made her feel worse than she had felt before, as she recognized that not only was her disagreement with her husband still unresolved, but now she also felt physically uncomfortable and ashamed of her actions.

7. In this last step you describe your plan to repair the harm that resulted from the problem behavior. This could involve describing what you will do to try to repair the blow to your self-confidence and/or the damage to a relationship(s) that the problem behavior caused. One helpful way to address the harm that resulted is to plan things that you can do differently next time. For example, look over what you circled as vulnerability factors and list ways to reduce them next time. Or think about ways to prevent the prompting event from happening again. The key in this step is to really open yourself to think about possible ways to make changes. Instead of dwelling on shame and remorse, use your commitment to stop binge eating to really let yourself think about small and big things you can do differently. It helps to write down the most realistic plans so that, when the time comes, you're more likely to access and use them. We strongly discourage any attempts to "repair" the binge by trying to make up for extra food eaten by eating less, exercising, vomiting, or any other compensatory behaviors. These will *not* repair the harm but instead will increase the likelihood that you will binge again, remaining locked in a vicious cycle of binge eating, restriction, and further binge eating.

Angela felt that to repair the harm she had done to herself she needed to renew her commitment to stop binge eating and to turn to this program first.

She felt it would have made an enormous difference if she had grabbed this book instead of her car keys! She made a specific plan to practice her skills and fill out her Diary Card every day. She also felt she had harmed her relationship with her husband and made a plan to apologize to him for how she had handled their disagreement.

Identifying Key Dysfunctional Links

Especially at the beginning stages of using Behavioral Chain Analysis Forms, you may find it difficult to identify the links (Step 4) that lead to a binge episode. In particular, it may be hard to identify the link that, for you, is the "point of no return"—the link (or links) at which you give up, or capitulate, and decide that there is no other option than to binge eat. An example of a key dysfunctional link might be feeling extremely agitated while thinking: "I have to treat myself with this chocolate! I won't deprive myself!" We call this type of link the "key dysfunctional link" to acknowledge that while the link has a powerful pull and certainly may *seem* true in the moment, you can later recognize how far you were from being in wise mind. For example, after the binge, it's clear that "depriving" yourself of the binge would actually have felt infinitely better than "treating" yourself in a way that inevitably left you filled with remorse.

The key dysfunctional links are often intense **F**eelings/emotions, but they can also be **C**ognitions/thoughts—or both. If you find a key dysfunctional link for a particular binge, mark it with an asterisk.

Angela marked as a key dysfunctional link the thought "I will feel better if I treat myself to some food." She felt it was when this thought entered her head that the idea of binge eating to manage the uncomfortable feelings about the disagreement with her husband took root and she started to think about which foods she could easily buy.

It wasn't that she had consciously made this link between feeling emotional pain and turning to food, but looking back she recognized that by this point she had started to shift away from the painful disagreement with her husband and was looking actively for a way to escape. Thoughts of food then led her to experience emotions such as desire, excitement, and anticipation—another key dysfunctional link that she identified. Though "positive," these emotions were certainly intense and felt highly uncomfortable—especially while she was trying to resist the urge to act on them.

While you can always break the behavioral chain at any link, you may find it is easier the earlier it is in the chain. The closer you are to the key dysfunctional link, the more difficult breaking the chain may feel. Angela sensed that, of all the places she could have broken a link, the easiest would have been when she was leaving her house. If she had practiced diaphragmatic breathing or had grabbed this book instead of (or along with) her other things and had started reading it, she may not have proceeded to the store.

Fortunately, Angela was still able to identify other skills to substitute to break her chain, even at her key dysfunctional links. For instance, she believed that if she had consulted her wise mind after having the thought that she would start to feel better if she treated herself to some of her favorite foods, she could have prevented herself from bingeing. Angela felt her wise mind would have helped her recall that she had never had a binge she hadn't ended up regretting. Her wise mind could also have gently asked her to try to picture how she would feel the next morning. Angela was sure that her wise mind would have helped her better manage this first key dysfunctional link.

Angela substituted another skill after she identified her second key dysfunctional link, experiencing desire and excitement about foods she would purchase. She believed she could have coped with these emotions by renewing the commitment to stop binge eating she had made in Chapter 2. Remembering how high a value she placed on stopping binge eating and finally having the chance to live the high-quality life she so desperately wanted would have made a huge difference in arresting her binge early in her behavioral chain.

To help you learn to identify your own key dysfunctional links, review how four different people filled out section 4 of the Behavioral Chain Analysis Form for a binge episode, shown on pages 95–96. These are typical of the types of links our patients have recorded as well as common key dysfunctional links. Each link is further categorized as an action, body sensation, cognition (thought), event, or feeling.

How Often and When Should You Fill Out a Behavioral Chain Analysis Form?

You may be wondering *how often* you should fill out your own Behavioral Chain Analysis Form. You can't do this too often, but start by filling one out in Exercise 1 and then filling out two this coming week as part of this chapter's homework (Exercise 4-A). This is important practice for filling out the form *at least* once a week as we ask you to do in coming chapters. (See the box at the end of the table of contents for information on printing out additional copies.) The more Behavioral Chain Analysis Forms you fill out, the more likely you'll be to use them to help you in the future.

You may also be wondering *when* to fill out a Behavioral Chain Analysis Form. It is important to fill it out as soon as possible after a binge. This will ensure more accurate information. Also, you do not have to wait until after a binge has occurred. You can carry a blank form around (or even jot the sequence down on a

Alejandro's Binge
with Key Dysfunctional Link(s)

4. Describe specific **links on chain**

I was in the mall and saw my favorite candy shop. _____ ABC(EF)

I felt a physical craving. _____ A(B)C-EF

I thought, "I can't resist them—they're too good!" _____ AB(C)EF

I experienced desire and some anxiety.*
KEY DYSFUNCTIONAL LINK _____ ABC-(EF)

I bought my favorite candy and chocolate and had a small binge in the car. _____ (A)BC-EF

Sheri's Binge with Key Dysfunctional Link(s)

4. Describe specific **links on chain**

I had a big argument with my partner. _____ ABC(EF)

I felt very angry and misunderstood. _____ ABC-(EF)

I thought: "I'll show her! I don't need her!"*
KEY DYSFUNCTIONAL LINK _____ AB(C)EF

I had a large binge at home on cereal and bread and butter. _____ (A)BC-EF

Mina's Binge with Key Dysfunctional Link(s)

4. Describe specific **links on chain**

I didn't get the raise I had expected. _____ ABC(EF)

I thought, "I didn't know this could hurt so much!" _____ AB(C)EF

I thought, "This is too much for me to take."*
KEY DYSFUNCTIONAL LINK _____ AB(C)EF

I felt hopeless and demoralized.*
KEY DYSFUNCTIONAL LINK _____ ABC-(EF)

When I got home I had a large binge on naan bread, rice, chicken tikka masala, and kheer. _____ (A)BC-EF

Michael's Binge with Key Dysfunctional Link(s)

4. Describe specific **links on chain**

I was at a buffet.	ABC(E)F
I saw a tempting dessert.	(A)BC-EF
I thought, "I should be able to eat what I want. It's not fair! Everyone else gets to."	AB(C)EF
I felt resentment and self-pity.* KEY DYSFUNCTIONAL LINK	ABC-(E)F
I had a large binge at the restaurant on multiple kinds of desserts.	(A)BC-EF

piece of paper or on your smartphone) *while* it is occurring. In other words, while you are experiencing the urge to binge, you can begin to analyze the links that led you to where you are. The act of slowing down and analyzing your behavior will help you to break the chain or at least give you a fighting chance.

EXERCISE 1   Behavioral Chain Analysis of Most Recent Binge

Choose your most recent binge and fill in the appropriate sections in the blank Behavioral Chain Analysis Form on page 97. Refer to the instructions starting on page 87. Use Angela's example on page 89 and the four binge examples with key dysfunctional links on pages 95–96 for help.

We remind you again that filling out Behavioral Chain Analysis Forms takes practice. Often several attempts are needed to get the hang of it. Obviously, the more of them you try to complete, the easier it will be to do them. And you might be pleasantly surprised at what you learn.

Note: It is **not** necessary to fill in every link in section 4 of the Behavioral Chain Analysis Form. Fill in only as many links as you need in order to describe what took place between the prompting event and your problem behavior. However, if you need more links than are provided, fill them out on a second sheet.

Chapter 4 Summary

This chapter focused on teaching you to become your own DBT coach, to be able to take a step back and learn from your past eating patterns so that you don't repeat them. To help you do this, we introduced you to the behavioral chain

Behavioral Chain Analysis Form

1. **Problem behavior** (include date took place _____):

   _____

2. **Prompting event:** _____

   _____

3. **Vulnerability factors** (circle and describe): physical illness, unbalanced sleep, intense emotional states, stressful environment, other:

   _____

4. Describe specific **links on chain** (and circle if **A**ction, **B**ody sensation, **C**ognition, **E**vent, or **F**eeling)

   5. Skillful behaviors to substitute

   _____ ABC-EF _____

   _____ ABC-EF _____

   _____ ABC-EF _____

   _____ ABC-EF _____

   _____ ABC-EF _____

   _____ ABC-EF _____

   _____ ABC-EF _____

   _____ ABC-EF _____

   _____ ABC-EF _____

   Mark the key dysfunctional link with an asterisk (*).

6. **What were the consequences of the behavior?**
   Immediate: _____

   _____

   Longer-term: _____

   _____

7. **Plan to repair harm and do things differently next time:**

   _____

   _____

analysis. This tool provides you with a structure for analyzing how a prompting event triggers a cascade of connected links that ultimately lead to a binge, which is followed by short- and longer-term consequences. Understanding these connections and what made you particularly vulnerable to them can help you do something different next time to prevent a binge. This involves using skills you have already learned from this program as well as new ones we will be teaching throughout the rest of the book. Instead of remaining stuck in destructive eating patterns, by the end of this program you will be fully equipped to practice and maintain the skillful behaviors you need for a healthy relationship with food.

Exercise 1 asks you to work through a Behavioral Chain Analysis Form using a recent binge-eating episode. If you had difficulty doing this, we strongly encourage you to go back and read through this chapter again. As you continue working through this program, you should continue to use the behavioral chain analysis tool.

Homework

Remember to check the box after you have completed each homework assignment.

HOMEWORK EXERCISE 4-A
Filling Out at Least Two Behavioral Chain Analyses

Over this next week, fill out at least **two Behavioral Chain Analysis Forms.** Do this as close in time as possible to when you had the problem behavior. It's a good idea to carry blank Behavioral Chain Analysis Forms with you. Remember that you do not need to worry about filling out the form perfectly or getting it exactly right. The most important thing is to gain practice using this tool! As you do, you will become more aware and in touch with your thoughts and feelings—something the invalidating environment did not encourage.

If you have difficulty filling out your chain, refer back to Angela's chain and the other examples, as well as the step-by-step instructions. Do your best to think of skillful behaviors to substitute, based on the skills you've learned so far or lessons learned from your past.

If you're having different types of problem behaviors (e.g., large binges, small binges, mindless eating), you might wonder which one you should choose as your problem behavior. Right now, we suggest not worrying too much about which problem behavior to prioritize—what is most important is getting experience using the chain. However, if further guidance would be helpful, refer to the discussion of the program goals and the four steps to getting the life you want in Chapter 3 on pages 62–65. Choose as your problem behavior the one that is closest to Step 1. For the example of experiencing large binges, small binges, and mindless eating, filling out your Behavioral Chain Analysis Form on any large binge episodes would take priority over small binges, which would take priority over mindless eating episodes.

If you are not having any types of binge episodes, you would fill out your Behavioral Chain Analysis Forms on other (nonbinge) eating-related problem behaviors such as emotional eating, mindless eating, or urges to binge.

❑ I have filled out at least two Behavioral Chain Analysis Forms this week.

❑ I have filled out my Diary Card daily.

❑ I have continued to use my wise mind this week, and if I find diaphragmatic breathing helpful, I have continued to practice it.

5

The Benefits of Dialectical
Thinking and Mindfulness

Remember in Chapter 1 when Leticia described going to her mother's home for dinner? She had planned to eat tiny portions of her favorite foods to stick to her "New Year's diet." Once she was there, smelling the tempting aromas, her desire felt so intense that she took extra servings, which broke her diet and led her to feel intense shame and disappointment in herself. At that point, Leticia's emotion mind reacted rigidly, based on a "black-and-white" logic that defines success as totally sticking to a diet. By this definition, she had already "failed" and might as well completely "blow" her diet, binge, and "start over" tomorrow. Emotion mind's perfectionistic thinking gave Leticia no other choices to consider.

We introduced Leticia to the skill of dialectical thinking to broaden her perspective and her future options, just as we want to help you broaden yours. Dialectal thinking involves holding two seemingly contradictory viewpoints *at the same time* by recognizing that there is always more than one way to view a situation, more than one way to solve a problem. Instead of a perfectionistic mindset that insists the "truth" is either black *or* white, a dialectical view sees the truth as encompassing black *and* white *and* all the infinite shades of gray that lie in between (see the spectrum depicted on page 101). Wise mind thinks dialectically.

In Leticia's case, we explained that her first task at her mother's dinner would have been to recognize that she was in emotion mind when she felt driven to binge because she had had the extra servings she had not planned for. Thinking dialectically, she could have said: "Yes, I did not stick to my New Year's diet, I feel disappointed and have an urge to totally blow it, *and* I am recommitting to my goals to not binge eat."

Dialectical thinking enables you to *have* a goal, such as honoring your commitment to stop binge eating, *and*, simultaneously, to *not meet* your goal. Dialectical

Black, white, and the shades of gray in between.

thinking allows success *and* failure to coexist. With dialectical thinking you don't have to abandon your goals if you don't meet them.

Leticia told us this way of thinking was not at all consistent with how she was raised. She was used to holding herself to the high standards her parents had set for her. She felt perfection was possible if she only tried hard enough. She didn't want to make excuses for anything less. However, the facts were that this mindset, in which there is only one way to do things and anything else is seen as failure, seemed to lead her to give up more and more easily. She found it very hard to motivate herself to persevere in the ways that truly difficult and complex tasks usually require. She constantly started over with new plans to "whip" herself into shape, although these new plans never seemed to work for very long before she slipped and felt defeated again. She admitted that "beating herself up" was not effective even though it was familiar. Although dialectical thinking likely feels unfamiliar, it offers you the freedom to fail and learn from your mistakes without judgment or self-punishment. Leticia's wise mind convinced her she could learn from her mistakes and move on. Ultimately, with practice, she found that dialectical thinking made it possible for her to "fail" and "succeed" at the same time.

A Dialectical View of the Commitment to Stop Binge Eating and Turn to This Program First

You can use dialectical thinking to help you keep your commitment to stop binge eating. In Chapter 2, you made a 100% commitment to hold in your mind and heart the truth that binge eating is incompatible with living the high-quality life you want. So on the one hand, you are absolutely committed to turning to the new skills you are learning in this program before you use food to numb uncomfortable emotions. Binge eating is not an option.

On the other hand, however, there is a second, seemingly contradictory truth that you must also hold in your mind and heart. If you do end up having a binge, you must accept yourself and not get stuck feeling like a failure. Change is hard, and none of us is perfect. If simply making a commitment to stop binge eating was all that was necessary to stop binge eating, you wouldn't need to learn all the skills we are teaching. You could have stopped reading at Chapter 2!

The dialectical view accepts that you are 100% committed to absolutely stopping binge eating *and* accepts that if you do binge, you will deal with the situation effectively by picking yourself up and returning to your 100% commitment. Dialectical thinking allows you to keep the commitment to abstinence even when you don't always meet your goal.

A good mental image to help you hold these two seemingly contradictory goals (e.g., aiming as high as possible *and* accepting/recommitting if you fall short) is an Olympic athlete. An Olympic athlete in training must focus only on winning and "going for the gold." This is the only mental state that makes it possible to reach such a challenging goal. If the Olympic-level athlete thought or said. "Aww, a bronze medal would be fine!" or "I'm just honored to be among such fine fellow athletes," his training mentality and performance would be compromised. Sports psychology has taught us the importance of vividly imagining your desired outcome and focusing exclusively on that.

But what happens if the Olympic athlete does not meet his goal? Let's say he's injured. The only effective choice is to accept this setback, try to learn from what happened, and try to prevent such an injury from happening again. This is an example of dialectical thinking—focusing on winning before the race but responding to a setback by brushing himself off, learning from it, and returning to a focus on the next race.

For a goal as important as stopping binge eating, which is *your* Olympic event, you must think like an Olympic athlete. You must commit to absolutely and totally living your life without using food in ways that ultimately cause you physical and psychological pain. Yet you must also be prepared for temporary failures. The key is to learn to fail well, which means accepting the binge, accepting yourself, and moving on. You create the synthesis that embodies dialectical thinking by recognizing that seemingly conflicting realities exist simultaneously—the reality of the binge and the reality of your commitment that binge eating is not an option.

At the same time, however, way, way in the back of your mind, so far back that you don't let it interfere with your focus on never binge eating again, is your knowledge that if you do binge, you will deal with it effectively and then return to your 100% commitment to stop binge eating from that point forward. This type of dialectical thinking about your commitment keeps you in the game, allowing you to use your "failures" to become more successful instead of becoming overwhelmed by your missteps.

A word of warning. Emotion mind can be tricky. Don't confuse dialectical thinking with rationalizing a binge. Sometimes, when you're experiencing a strong urge to binge, emotion mind can say that it's OK to give in to your urge to binge because you can just start again tomorrow. This is not something that your wise mind, which wants what is truly in your best interests in the long run, would say. Only emotion mind would ever give you permission to binge.

Dealing with Binge-Eating Setbacks Using Dialectical Thinking

John had always seen himself as a black-and-white thinker but was surprised to learn how his black-and-white thinking could have such a big influence on his behavior, particularly his difficulty stopping binge eating. John found himself needing to reread the section about dialectical thinking several times. In doing so, he made an important discovery. He realized he actually did have a lot of experience with thinking dialectically, but it wasn't when he was thinking about his own actions—it was when he was thinking about his friends. For instance, John was able to see his friends as hardworking, and he could value their efforts even if they didn't always get the results (like a bonus) that they had hoped for. He could validate their frustration and disappointment without condemning them as whiners or failures. Over time, and with practice, John was able to use this more flexible approach with his own situations, which reduced his tendency to be so critical when he experienced setbacks with binge eating. For example, instead of saying to himself, "I haven't been spending enough time doing the homework for this program—no wonder I'm still overeating!" he practiced saying, "I haven't been spending as much time on the homework in this program as I had planned" and "I can take a few minutes now to read some more and keep going."

EXERCISE 1 Practicing Shifting from Rigid to Dialectical Thinking

Think of times you typically get stuck at a "point of no return." These are the times when your emotion mind pushes you toward black-and-white or rigid, perfectionistic thinking. For Leticia, this "point of no return" is often after she has eaten something unplanned and her emotion mind says: "I can't stand it that I already messed up, so I have to binge." To practice dialectical thinking, she needed to step back and, like John, think about what she might say to encourage a friend or loved one facing a similar situation. She would never judge them for "messing up" and tell them their only option was to binge.

We suggested she use dialectical thinking to stretch her mind by using "and" between seemingly contradictory viewpoints, allowing failure and success to coexist. Practicing dialectical thinking, Leticia could say: "Yes I messed up and ate more than I'd planned **and** I will feel so much better tomorrow by recommitting right now to stopping binge eating." Or "I can feel bad **and** not have to make myself feel even worse by to continuing to overeat." Or "This is my opportunity to be like an Olympic athlete by falling **and** getting right back up."

Practice applying dialectical thinking to one or two things your emotion mind tells you that typically push you toward rigid thinking and a "point of no return." Start by writing down what your emotion mind says to you. Then use dialectical thinking by adding an "**and**" to help you develop a flexible mindset. (Note: Homework Exercise 5-A provides additional opportunities to practice dialectical thinking to help you shift out of your emotion mind's rigid, perfectionistic mindset.)

1. **Emotion Mind:**

_____

_____

   Dialectical Thinking:

_____

_____

   and _____

_____

2. **Emotion Mind:**

_____

_____

   Dialectical Thinking:

_____

_____

   and _____

_____

Kat wrote:

Emotion Mind: *I messed up and ate more chocolate truffles than I planned, so I might as well just binge on all of them and start over tomorrow.*

Dialectical Thinking: *Yes, I feel very disappointed that I broke my plan, and I don't have to make myself feel even worse by giving up on myself and continuing to binge eat.*

Using Dialectical Thinking to Accept Yourself and Decide to Change

Another useful way to apply dialectical thinking involves developing a more flexible view of yourself. For example, you started this program because you recognized you had to make changes to fully live up to your potential. However, you also must accept yourself as you are right in this moment. Otherwise, you risk putting yourself into a state of self-criticism, self-loathing, and self-aversion—a state in which it's very easy to feel hopeless, give up, and binge eat. A dialectical view asks you to change while accepting yourself exactly as you are in this moment.

The key to being able to do this is to realize that accepting yourself does not require that you approve of where you are or like it. This means accepting yourself in the same way that you already accept gravity. If you push a tissue box off a table, it will fall to the floor. Gravity simply *is*. You accept the force of gravity without getting stuck in whether you approve or disapprove of it. This allows you to move effectively in the world. Similarly, you can experience your physical appearance, your weight, the consequences you have suffered due to how you have treated your body over the years as facts that, *at this moment,* are forces that make up reality—just like gravity. Accepting them because they simply *are,* instead of getting stuck in approval or disapproval, allows you to get unstuck from self-loathing and make the changes in your life you want to make. Just as a rocket scientist has to take gravity into consideration to successfully launch a spacecraft, you have to accept all of who you are in the present moment to launch a new set of behaviors that will enable you to create a binge-free life.

On the one hand you have committed to change because you are dissatisfied with your current reality. On the other hand, you are accepting yourself exactly as you are *in this moment* so you can change. This is the dialectic. These two views coexist because they are true at the same time—even though they seem contradictory. This is the *synthesis.* Accepting yourself as you are in this moment, without judgment, is likely something you have never been able to do. Being able to do this—to even be able to think about doing it—means you *have already begun to change.*

Some people may find it helpful to think of the words in the Serenity Prayer: "God, grant me the serenity to accept the things I cannot change; the courage to change the things I can; and wisdom to know the difference."

EXERCISE 2 Applying Dialectical Thinking to Accept Yourself and Change

This exercise is intended to give you practice in applying dialectical thinking in instances when becoming stuck in negative and unhelpful self-judgments about yourself increases your emotional discomfort and hence your vulnerability to binge eating. Examples of negative self-judgments might include concerns about your body's current weight or shape, how your clothes fit, or food choices you've made today or over the past few days.

Use the space below to practice applying dialectical thinking by identifying one or two things your emotion mind typically tells you that tend to push you into a state of negative and unhelpful self-judgment. Then apply dialectical thinking by adding an "and" to help you acknowledge what you need to accept. This allows you to shift from being stuck in your negative self-judgments and move ahead toward achieving your long-term goals. (Note: Homework Exercise 5-A offers additional opportunities to apply dialectical thinking to help you shift out of an unhelpful spiral of negative self-judgment when you are dissatisfied with your current reality.)

1. **Emotion Mind:**

   _____

   _____

   Dialectical Thinking:

   _____

   _____

   and _____

   _____

2. **Emotion Mind:**

   _____

   _____

   Dialectical Thinking:

   _____

   _____

   and _____

   _____

Kat wrote:

Emotion Mind: *My husband doesn't find me attractive anyway. I deserve at least to eat what I want.*

Dialectical Thinking: *I can feel angry at him and unloved <u>and</u> I can still not binge.*

> **Emotion Mind:** *Recently, every dress I tried looked so awful I wanted to binge because it's hopeless to try.*
>
> **Dialectical Thinking:** *I can feel disappointed and hopeless about my appearance and want to binge <u>and</u> I can want to have a high-quality, highly satisfying life. Binge eating will just make me feel worse.*

Accepting Contradictory Feelings about Stopping Binge Eating

Another situation where dialectical thinking is useful involves tolerating the part of you that wants to eat as much as you want *and* the part of you that sincerely wants to stop binge eating. Binge eating has likely been a main coping strategy for you when life has felt too difficult to manage. It absolutely makes sense that while you want to stop binge eating, actually having to live without the comfort food can bring might trigger emotions like fear, sadness, loss, deprivation, anxiety, anger, and/or a sense of injustice. It's perfectly normal to be ambivalent about stopping binge eating or attempting anything that's difficult and requires a great deal of effort. Dialectical thinking can help you flexibly acknowledge and accept your ambivalent feelings so they can coexist. Accepting ambivalence instead of struggling against it will make stopping binge eating easier.

For example, let's return to Leticia's story. As we continued to explore what took place that evening, Leticia was able to remember more details than she had originally recalled. This is common. Initially, all she had remembered was experiencing intense desire, eating extra helpings, and not being able to cope with having broken her original plan. But now she remembered that even before she served herself the extra food, she noticed her mouth watering. She remembered feeling upset and self-critical for even desiring extra food because she did not want to desire anything she had already decided she wasn't going to eat. She hated having to set limits with herself. She wanted to *want* to stay on her food plan, and anything else was intolerable. Her emotion mind said: "You're going to have to give in and have more! It's too hard to want something and not have it! This will work only if you're happy with the small amounts you're supposed to have!"

From this point forward, Leticia can use dialectical thinking to help her in such instances. Applying dialectical thinking, she could say to herself: "Of course I want to eat more, and that's OK! I can want to eat more, *and* I can want even more than that to feel good about myself tomorrow by not binge eating. "

It's important to point out that it's also possible for you to get stuck in black-and-white thinking that is driven solely by your reasonable mind. While being stuck in emotion mind's rigid thinking is what we usually hear about, it's also common for some people, when they feel self-critical about their binge eating, to swing to the other side of the continuum and think only about what is "logical" or "rational"—without paying any attention to the validity of their emotions. For example, imagine that after Leticia had binged—having given in to her emotion mind's insistence that setting any limits was impossible if she experienced any struggle with desiring more than she had decided to have—Leticia's reasonable mind tells her that she should skip breakfast and lunch the next day to compensate for the excess calories.

Unfortunately, attempts to think "purely" in terms of logic and rationality can feel invalidating to our sensitive emotion mind. While Leticia's plan might work upon occasion, focusing too intensely on reasonable mind forces her emotion mind to "scream" louder to be heard, which increases the probability she will turn to binge eating. For example, when she skips breakfast and lunch the next day, she is more likely to be hungry and irritable by the afternoon and therefore more vulnerable to her emotion mind and thus to overeating—which perpetuates the cycle of binge eating. Dialectical thinking can help Leticia accept that she didn't follow her plan *and* that restricting herself by cutting calories is not an effective "fix."

EXERCISE 3 Accepting Contradictory Feelings about Stopping Binge Eating

The purpose of this exercise is give you a chance to practice applying dialectical thinking in instances when you are experiencing ambivalent or contradictory feelings about giving up binge eating.

Use the space below to identify one or two things your emotion mind and reasonable mind typically say (or what you recall from the past) when you are feeling pulled to binge eat or are feeling ambivalent about giving up binge eating. Then follow this with dialectical thinking by adding an "and" to help you acknowledge and accept these contradictory feelings.

1. **Emotion Mind:**

_____

_____

Rational Mind:

_____

_____

Dialectical Thinking:

_____

_____

and _____

_____

2. **Emotion Mind:**

_____

_____

Rational Mind:

_____

_____

Dialectical Thinking:

_____

_____

and _____

_____

Kat wrote:

Emotion Mind: *Everyone else will be having lots of desserts! It's not fair that I don't get to!*

Reasonable Mind: *You shouldn't be comparing what you eat to what others eat.*

Dialectical Thinking: *It's natural to want to be like everyone else, <u>and</u> even though life's not fair I will feel good tomorrow for keeping my commitment to myself.*

Emotion Mind: *I wasn't planning to eat this, but it's just too hard not to.*

Rational Mind: *It doesn't matter that it's hard; it's not on your plan, so don't eat it.*

Dialectical Thinking: *I have strong urges that are important to acknowledge, <u>and</u> I can tolerate feeling the difficulty.*

Be gentle. Commitment to making changes in your best interests is an active process. It involves continual awareness—commitment and recommitment—over and over.

As you continue to practice dialectical thinking you will find it easier to accept yourself as you are and simultaneously accept the fact that you deserve to be free of binge eating!

Introduction to the Mindfulness Skill "Observing"

The next mindfulness skill, *observing,* involves learning to have an experience without getting caught up in it, judging it, or reacting to it. This requires learning to step back and detach from your experiences. A useful image to have is to think of yourself as a recording device. You are simply taking in information without labeling it. It is as if your eyes are a video camera and your ears a recorder. Like these devices, you want to observe without evaluating or reacting to the information you take in. You can decide where to place the recording device but not what information your senses detect. You can also practice observing by imagining yourself as having a "nonstick" mind, just like a nonstick frying pan. You are not holding on to experiences or pushing them away. You are simply noticing what is taking place without getting stuck in or trying to control what you experience.

The skill of observing is very useful for helping you get unstuck from being in your emotion mind and accessing your wise mind more easily. Since emotion mind is the state of mind in which binge eating takes place, being able to shift out of emotion mind into wise mind is crucial. The box on the facing page describes Angela's experience with practicing observing to reduce her urges to binge eat.

Try the following exercise to practice the skill of observing and cultivate your ability to be a wise and nonreactive observer of events.

EXERCISE 4   An Experiential Exercise to Introduce Observing

"Begin by putting both feet on the floor. Focus your awareness on your feet, just observing the experience of your feet on the floor. You are just turning your attention there, not describing the experience of your feet on the floor. You are practicing noticing the experience without anything else—without words or judgment. Just observing, cultivating a focused awareness.

"Now focus your awareness on the muscles in your neck and shoulders. Just observe the experience, the sensations without words. Just keep your attention there—stepping back from the experience, being aware of it."

Observing means that you are allowing yourself to experience an awareness of the moment, no matter what is happening. Observing an experience does not mean trying to change it or attempting to stop or end it.

Using Observing with Your Emotions

You can also use observing with your emotions. For example, if you want to practice observing sadness, you would allow the sadness to be there as part of the moment, without trying to change it, make it different, or run from it. You can

Angela's Practice of Observing

Angela had long recognized that her tendency to become overwhelmed by emotions was a trigger for her binges. The skill of observing helped her learn how to bring a moment of emotional detachment to situations so that she was more aware of her feelings and could react accordingly. This also helped reduce her anxiety, as she was often worrying about things that hadn't happened yet. It was easy for Angela to forget to use observing and get wrapped up in situations; however, she did find that practice helped a lot, and she became increasingly skilled at observing emotionally loaded situations without judgment. This helped her identify when she was in emotion mind and shift into wise mind. Observing helped create a sense of an internal "pause." She felt particularly proud of herself one day at work when she was furious at her boss and felt strong urges to binge on her drive home. Instead, before she left, she practiced observing with a print hanging in her office—simply noticing the colors and shapes in front of her while breathing from her diaphragm. Doing this helped her access her wise mind, which reminded her of how important her commitment to stop binge eating was. She decided to talk over the situation with a trusted colleague and got useful advice without harming herself with food.

practice observing any emotion—anger, anxiety, joy, and so on. If you don't know what the emotion is, you can observe physical sensations like shallow breathing, clammy hands, or a pounding heart, or notice that your face feels hot.

It's important to remember that observing is separate from the experience itself. Your heart beating and the act of noticing that your heart is beating are two separate phenomena. Your heart is always beating whether you are noticing it or not. You can observe your thinking, which is different from the act of thinking. The same is true with emotions. Observing or watching your emotions is different from experiencing the emotions themselves. Indeed you probably have emotions going on that you may not be aware of.

Observing your life as it is unfolding is similar to being in the eye of a hurricane, with emotions swirling all around you. Observing offers you a calm center into which you can step to watch and maintain awareness without getting caught up in the storm.

As we mentioned, observing is an important skill you can use to interrupt yourself if you feel you are on the path to a binge-eating episode. It can help you stay in the moment, observing your experience—including your external surroundings as well as your internal thoughts and emotions—instead of being swept along by them. This can help you avoid getting stuck in emotion mind's judgments that serve as links on your behavioral chain toward a binge. Concentrating on what is happening in the present can also help you act more effectively to break links in the present instead of remaining stuck in anxiety about future events.

Chapter 5 Summary

In this chapter we introduced two new skills: dialectical thinking and observing. Dialectical thinking means getting away from black-and-white thinking, where you are either 100% "successful" or 100% "unsuccessful." It involves recognizing that with every thought or position, an opposing thought or position is possible. An example we discussed several times is how you have made a 100% commitment to stop binge eating. Anything less is selling yourself short. But at the same time, you need to be prepared for a slip so that if it does occur, you can learn from it. Conflicting forces and thoughts will always occur. Dialectical thinking involves the ability to recognize and accept them. Another valuable way to use dialectical thinking involves accepting who you are at this moment, while at the same time accepting that you want to change. A third way to apply dialectical thinking is toward accepting conflicting feelings about giving up binge eating. The exercises in this chapter were intended to help you practice applying dialectical thinking.

We also discussed using the skill of observing. Observing involves just noticing an experience without getting caught up, judging, or reacting to it. As we will discuss in the homework section, you should start to practice observing with physical sensations. As you become more comfortable with this skill, you can use it to observe your emotions. Observing emotions involves experiencing the emotion you are feeling without judging it or yourself. The chapter includes an experiential exercise to practice observing.

This program puts you in the driver's seat. We teach you different skills so that you can decide how best and in what situations to use them. If at this point you don't feel confident with a certain concept or idea, we suggest you go back and review it. Congratulations on your progress so far!

Homework

Remember to check the box after you have completed each homework assignment.

HOMEWORK EXERCISE 5-A
Creating a Dialectical Thinking Card

As you did in Chapter 2, copy some of what you wrote above for the three dialectical thinking exercises (Exercises 1–3 in this chapter) onto a small card that you can carry in your wallet or purse (using either a 3" × 5" index card or a piece of folded paper). Look at the card and practice dialectical thinking by reading over your answers to the exercises at least once a day. In addition, be on the lookout for the following three types of situations where you can practice dialectical thinking to prevent a binge: (1) when your emotion mind's rigid, perfectionistic mindset tells you that you have "failed" because you have eaten more than you had planned; (2) when you are dissatisfied with your current reality and want to shift out of an unhelpful spiral of negative self-judgment and self-loathing; and (3) when you are struggling against, rather than accepting, your ambivalent feelings about your commitment to stop binge eating.

❑ I have copied my writing about dialectical thinking onto a card I can keep with me so that I can look at it each day and also when I have an urge to binge.

HOMEWORK EXERCISE 5-B

Practicing Observing over the Coming Week

Practice observing once every day over the next week. Start by observing physical sensations. For example, practice observing the sensations of your feet on the floor, the sense of temperature through your hands as they rest on a table, the physical sounds you hear while sitting reading this book, what your eyes take in as you look out a window, the taste of toothpaste as you brush your teeth, and so forth. When you feel ready, move on to observing emotions. In the space below, describe your experiences practicing this skill over the week.

_____

_____

_____

_____

_____

_____

❑ I have practiced the skill of observing once every day this week.

❑ I have filled out my Diary Card daily.

❑ I have filled out at least one Behavioral Chain Analysis Form this week.

❑ I have used the skills I find most helpful so that I can use my wise mind and stop binge eating before it happens.

6

Becoming a More
Skillful Observer

John, like many of our patients, was often very judgmental toward himself. He carried a deep sense of shame, feeling he didn't measure up to others' expectations. His long-standing difficulty with binge eating was one area in which he judged himself negatively, but his judgments encompassed almost every major aspect of his life. He constantly compared himself negatively to his coworkers despite being a successful executive. He worried that his colleagues disliked him and that his friends thought he was sloppy and had low standards because he was overweight. On the rare occasions when he entertained at home, he worried that his guests thought he was a poor host. As for his parents, he actually knew what their judgments were because they frequently called him selfish and self-involved for rarely visiting them. John's shame and anxiety were easily triggered. He was especially self-critical and vulnerable to binge eating after any interaction with others.

For John, therefore, the skill we call adopting a nonjudgmental stance was particularly helpful. As John learned about this skill, he began to notice just how often he judged himself. And instead of judging his judging, he practiced accepting that he was a person who very much wanted others to think well of him. His wise mind said that criticizing himself when he was uncertain about others' reactions was easier than accepting that he didn't always have control over how people responded to him. This helped him feel greater compassion for himself, which, in turn, made it easier for him to practice the skill of adopting a nonjudgmental stance and rephrase critical thoughts into less judgmental ones. For example, he became aware how often after a business dinner he would rehash what had taken place, especially moments when he felt awkward: "I sounded so stupid! Mario [John's boss] looked uncomfortable the whole time. He probably wanted me to just shut up." John would try to step back, just observing the facts, and say something like "There were times during the dinner when I didn't speak as clearly as I would have wished. I'm feeling ashamed. I feel like my boss noticed and felt ashamed for me, but I actually don't know if that is true. I know I was doing my best, but it might have helped if I had used some diaphragmatic breathing to be calmer. I'll try that next time." Initially, he frequently noticed and rephrased judgmental thoughts. Over time and with practice, he found he made fewer and fewer of these negative judgments about himself. Often he simply needed to breathe deeply to feel calmer and less judgmental.

Adopting a Nonjudgmental Stance

How do you respond when you've done something you've disapproved of? We've heard many patients refer to themselves as "stupid" or as "acting like an idiot" after they've made a mistake, call themselves "disgusting" after they felt they ate too much, or say they are "stupid" to be reacting with hurt to something someone said to them. These are examples of judgments and pretty harsh ones!

But of course some kinds of judgments can be useful. For example, judgments allow us to make decisions quite quickly. Sometimes these quick decisions can be protective—like when we take a quart of milk out of the fridge and discover from a quick sniff that it has gone "bad." Deciding that the milk is "bad" involves making a judgment. The judgment, "bad," really means that the milk has been spoiled by bacteria, and it is associated with feeling disgust or revulsion. Disgust protects us from drinking the milk and getting sick. Judging the milk as "bad" means we don't have to think about the situation in great detail. The judgment ("bad") is associated with an emotion (disgust) that carries an instruction ("don't drink") that protects us.

In situations where no immediate action is needed to keep us safe, however, negative self-judgments can create a vicious cycle. Calling yourself "stupid" or "disgusting" leads to self-loathing, shame, and other painful emotions that make you more vulnerable to binge eating as an attempt to temporarily escape these feelings. Then, if you do binge, you have to deal with additional negative self-judgments about bingeing—exacerbating your shame and setting you up to binge again.

Adopting a nonjudgmental stance means not judging or labeling your binge eating as *bad* or yourself as a *bad* person for binge eating (or a *good* person for not doing so). The issue at stake is not a moral one. Binge eating makes you feel ashamed, wastes time, energy, and money, and inevitably leads to feeling miserable. The point is to stop the vicious cycle of the good–bad, right–wrong battle and instead just observe the consequences in terms of their effect on your self-esteem, physical health, and life goals.

Another problem with judging is that our judgments often masquerade as facts. For example, the statement "I am overweight" may be a fact. But if it implies the judgment "Being overweight is bad and overweight people are less worthy than normal-weight or thin people," then the judging piggybacks on the otherwise factual statement.

The mindfulness skill of adopting a nonjudgmental stance asks you to take the time to observe and describe yourself and your behaviors without activating emotions like disgust, shame, or hopelessness that would lead you to act quickly or impulsively from your emotion mind. Instead of labeling someone or something as good or bad, right or wrong, valuable or not, worthwhile or worthless, you take the time to describe what or who is being evaluated in terms of its consequences. For example, if you say to yourself, "I am a bad parent because I snapped at my child," you are likely to feel ashamed. Adopting a nonjudgmental stance and focusing on the consequences of your behavior, you might say: "Snapping at my child hurt his feelings, which I don't want to do, and I would like to change this behavior." The first sentence is a judgment, while the second sentence emphasizes the consequences of the behavior and what you want to change.

Imagine that you've just made yourself a cup of coffee. After you taste it, you tell yourself that it's "bad." How could that information help you improve the next cup of coffee you make? You'd need to slow down and describe your experience in terms of whether it was too bitter, too hot, too watery, or too sweet. Only this type of detailed information can help you make the changes you need to make to increase the likelihood of making the next cup of coffee more to your liking.

We understand that it's the nature of our minds to compare things, evaluate, and judge. Yet quick negative self-judgments (e.g., "I'm a failure, I'm no good, I'm a disgrace, I'm an embarrassment") are destructive and can become so pervasive that you may not be aware that you're using them. For example, you may find yourself feeling depressed "for no particular reason" and not be aware of how your emotions were triggered by an episode of negative self-judging.

Practicing adopting a nonjudgmental stance toward your experience and what comes up in your mind will help increase your awareness of the amount of judging that you do. Try not to judge yourself when you find yourself judging! It is very difficult to change the tendency to make negative snap judgments. When you catch yourself judging, try to simply observe your judgments.

The skill of adopting a nonjudgmental stance may sound abstract, but once you get the hang of it, understanding how to use it becomes easier. The following exercise offers a useful image to help you practice.

EXERCISE 1 Observing Judgments on a Conveyor Belt

Try to imagine that the thoughts in your mind are like luggage coming down an airport conveyor belt. When you see your judgmental piece of "luggage," practice observing the judgments. It can be helpful to "wave" at your judgment, acknowledging that "Yes, there's that judgment again." For example, you might note to yourself: "Hello again, judgment about the shape of my body" or "Yes, there's that judgment I have about binge eating." Much like a piece of luggage on a conveyor belt, your judgmental thought may circle around repeatedly in your brain. Remember that mindfulness is like a muscle and you may have to observe your judgment again and again before you can let it go.

Try this now: Practice observing your current thoughts for a few minutes as if they are on a conveyor belt. Are there any judgmental pieces of luggage? What is it like to practice observing them while attempting to adopt a nonjudgmental stance? Write about your experience below.

_____

_____

_____

_____

_____

_____

_____

Kat wrote:

After I closed my eyes and started observing my thoughts, I immediately started noticing that I had judgments about how I wasn't doing this exercise correctly. I observed telling myself, as I often do, "This is too hard. I can't do it. I'm terrible at visualizations." I tried to step back and put that thought on the conveyor belt and watch it as it disappeared around the corner. As soon as it left it seemed to come right back. I tried waving at it and imagined it as our familiar beat-up red suitcase. "See you, judgment!" For a moment, I noticed I felt more calm and less worried about doing this perfectly.

It is possible to express preferences, values, or emotions without adding judgment. For example, the statement "I like jazz better than country music" is a preference, not a problematic judgment. Judgments such as "this is better than that" can have their place in providing feedback (e.g., grades) or information about what to continue, change, or stop. The difficulty is when the judgment is presented as a statement of fact, or moral certainty, such as saying that jazz *is better* than country music.

Negative self-judging is a kind of self-invalidation. Many people with a history of binge eating have difficulty validating (nonjudgmentally accepting) themselves and their feelings. In fact, they often seem to invalidate themselves automatically, or mindlessly, without awareness. Self-invalidation and negative self-judgments can be thought of as stomping all over your experience, including your feelings, thoughts, and actions. Instead of invalidating yourself, practice observing the contents of your mind. If you notice a judgment, label it as a judgment and let it go down the conveyor belt (as in Exercise 1). This will bring awareness to the otherwise automatic link between self-judging and its consequences.

EXERCISE 2   Practicing Adopting a Nonjudgmental Stance

Write down statements you make to yourself that involve taking a judgmental stance. Practice restating these judgments in neutral terms that emphasize observation, understanding, and corrective action. Focus especially on those judgments that may be linked to your binge eating.

   This exercise is something you can use throughout this program and afterward to help you stop making ineffective negative or snap judgments about yourself or others.

1. **Judgmental Stance:**

   _____

   _____

   Nonjudgmental Stance:

   _____

   _____

   _____

   _____

2. **Judgmental Stance:**

   _____

   _____

Nonjudgmental Stance:

_____

_____

_____

_____

3. **Judgmental Stance:**

_____

_____

Nonjudgmental Stance:

_____

_____

_____

_____

Kat wrote:

1. **Judgmental Stance:** _It is awful that I binge ate. I have no willpower._

   Nonjudgmental Stance: _I had a binge-eating episode because I became upset and didn't use any of the skills I learned in this program. I will write out a Behavioral Chain Analysis Form and see what I could have done differently._

2. **Judgmental Stance:** _I am a mean person for being angry at my friend for canceling her visit at the last minute._

   Nonjudgmental Stance: _I was looking forward to my friend's visit and had put in a lot of effort to prepare for it. My feelings of anger and disappointment are valid. I do not have to express these feelings to her if I don't feel it would be effective, but I don't have to pretend to myself that I don't feel them._

3. **Judgmental Stance:** _I look horribly awful in this outfit. I am a fat pig._

   Nonjudgmental Stance: _I may not look the way I want to look right now, but I'm doing my best to live the life I want to and get my eating under control. And for right now, that is enough._

Focusing on One Thing in the Moment

Focusing on one thing in the moment is the skill of learning to control your attention. The essence of this skill is acting with undivided attention, bringing the whole of your person to bear on the present activity whether it is eating, driving, listening, or thinking about a problem. Focusing on one thing in the moment is the opposite of multitasking. It involves being fully present in the moment you are in, bringing your full awareness to the current moment's activity without letting your attention wander to something else. Focusing on one thing in the moment also involves becoming aware of those moments when your mind wanders and then bringing your mind and attention back to the present moment.

Focusing on one thing in the moment has to do with concentration, being able to stay focused. Brushing your teeth while focusing on one thing in the moment means just brushing your teeth. It means trying to stay in the moment. When you try to anticipate the future or ruminate about the past, you miss out on what is happening in the present, in this moment. Life, after all, is only a series of moments.

Practicing focusing on one thing in the moment takes patience to concentrate and remain in the present moment. Impatience is tapping your foot, wanting to get out of this moment, wanting to move on. Patience is letting things be as they are in the moment, focusing on one thing in the moment. So, when you practice focusing on one thing in the moment, think of the experience of being patient and of letting go. Waiting in line can be turned from an inconvenience to an opportunity to concentrate on the moment and practice observing while focusing on one thing in the moment. You can also practice focusing on one thing in the moment while paying attention to your breath during diaphragmatic breathing.

EXERCISE 3   Practicing Focusing on One Thing in the Moment

In this exercise, we are asking you to focus on your breath and only your breath coming in and out of your nostrils for 30–60 seconds. If you notice that your attention wanders, gently adopt a nonjudgmental stance and bring your focus back to the task at hand, which is simply observing your breath. After you have practiced this, describe your experience practicing the skill of focusing on one thing in the moment below.

_____

_____

_____

———————————————————————————

———————————————————————————

———————————————————————————

Kat wrote:

I started out being able to focus my attention on my breathing and only my breathing pretty well, at least at first. But then I found myself distracted by the rise and fall of my stomach. I practiced adopting a non-judgmental stance and said: "It's OK. There's nothing I can do about my stomach right now" and gently brought my attention back to my breathing. Although I had to keep bringing my attention back to my breath a few times, it felt like it got easier.

Being Effective

This next mindfulness skill, being effective, involves focusing on doing what works. When you practice this skill, you are concentrating on achieving your goal, not on "being right" or "being perfect." Being effective means playing with the cards you have been dealt. It's playing by the rules—whether or not you like them.

Being effective is the opposite of "cutting off your nose to spite your face." In other words, being effective means that at times you have to give in instead of insisting that things go the way you want them to go. Digging in your heels and insisting that things go a certain way can propel you into emotion mind and into binge eating.

You *may* be right; your way might indeed *be* the fair way. But when you rigidly adhere to something other than the present reality, things just will not work. Being effective requires accepting reality as it is whether or not it's the way you think it should be. It means accepting that things aren't always fair.

Imagine what would happen if you visited a busy city to do some shopping and decided that because people *should* be trustworthy, you *shouldn't* have to lock your car and you *should* be able to leave packages you just bought on the car seat while going for a walk in a nearby park. If your goal is to take your purchases home, regardless of whether it is right or wrong if your packages are stolen, deciding not to lock your car is simply not being effective.

Being effective means keeping your focus on your goals. As part of this program, your goal is to stop binge eating. Instead of insisting that you should be able to have a high-quality life and continue to binge eat, being effective means accepting (as you did in Chapter 2) that binge eating is simply not an effective way to manage emotional pain. What *is* being effective is learning and practicing the skills taught in this program. Being effective means staying in touch with your wise mind and being mindful of consequences.

You may be wondering how you will know when to use being effective. One clue that you should use this skill is finding yourself thinking that a situation "just isn't fair!" Instead, ask yourself what your objective in the situation is and then practice being effective and focus on what actions are needed to achieve your goals.

> Leticia told us that she had made progress with her binge eating, but one of the remaining prompting events continued to be going to her mother's home for family meals. These dinners were very important to her mother, who was very proud of her traditional southern cooking skills and very much wanted her entire family present. Leticia struggled with whether or not she should skip these events because more often than not she ended up overeating even when she didn't binge. It seemed that there was almost no way to participate in these occasions without taking in more food than she felt good about or her body needed. She was angry that her mother cared so much about these dinners and that her brothers and sisters all seemed comfortable with them. She was also angry that she wasn't thinner so that indulging once in a while wouldn't have much of an effect on her body.
>
> Leticia was so upset and focused on the unfairness of the situation that she wanted to avoid the dinners altogether.

Choosing to practice being effective meant Leticia had to shift her focus from the unfairness of the situation to identifying her objective. When Leticia focused on how important it was for her to be with her family and not how unfair the situation was, she felt calmer and more willing to attend the dinners and deal with the current realities of her situation.

EXERCISE 4   Understanding Being Effective

a. **Think of a time when you were focused on the unfairness of a situation** or how you hoped things would be a certain way—rather than accepting the reality of the situation. **How might this have led to binge eating?** Write about it below.

_____

_____

Kat wrote:

When I found out that one of my best friends was diagnosed with dementia, it was shocking and devastating. She was like a second mother to me, and the thought of losing her was intolerable and felt completely unfair. I couldn't stand the idea of seeing her, and so I stayed away. This made me feel like a terrible friend and led me to binge.

b. Looking back now, **write about how the experience would have been different if you had accepted the realities of the situation.**

Kat wrote:

I regret that I wasted those weeks avoiding her and turning to food when I could have been spending time with her. If I had accepted the reality of the situation, I would have seen that what I really wanted was to be a good friend and be with her. I've been able to do that since but only after a lot of wasted time and needless binge eating.

Chapter 6 Summary

This chapter focused on three skills that will help you access your wise mind. Each of these skills is about focusing on the present moment and getting the most out of it. The first skill, adopting a nonjudgmental stance, is about not being judgmental when you are observing yourself and your behaviors. It's about avoiding negative self-judgments, such as evaluating yourself in moral terms (e.g., good or bad). Instead, adopting a nonjudgmental stance involves evaluating yourself and your behaviors in terms of observing, understanding, and corrective action. We also discussed how judging often occurs automatically, without self-awareness. You will have plenty of opportunities to practice catching yourself whenever you notice you are making a negative self-judgment.

The second skill discussed was focusing on one thing in the moment. This skill involves bringing your full attention to the task at hand. Although the concept may seem simple, it is often the opposite of what we are used to. Multitasking has become normal for most people even though research has shown that multitasking is actually less effective than doing tasks one at a time. Focusing on one thing in the moment involves *focusing your full attention on the one thing you are doing, the one moment you are in.* Focusing on one thing in the moment can be very helpful to stop the binge-eating cycle by bringing your full attention to what you are doing at a particular moment.

The final skill discussed is being effective. Being effective is about making the most of your current situation rather than focusing on how things *should* be or how you would like them to be. This skill is about playing the cards you have been dealt. Being effective can be very useful when you find yourself upset about the injustice of a situation or when you are unsure about how to get what you want. Being effective involves looking at the real options and real limitations you have and then deciding how you can act most skilfully within those limitations.

Homework

Remember to check the box after you have completed each homework assignment.

HOMEWORK EXERCISE 6-A

Practice Adopting a Nonjudgmental Stance over the Coming Week

Take a moment to ask yourself how judging operates in your life. In the space provided, try to answer the following questions: Does judging play a role in the chain of events that lead you to binge eat? Is it a key dysfunctional link? If so, how can you start using the skill of adopting a nonjudgmental stance this week? This can be as simple as writing down the judgmental stance you noticed and rewriting the nonjudgmental alternative, as in Exercise 2. You can then refer to the nonjudgmental stance whenever you have the judgmental one. For additional practice with adopting a nonjudgmental stance, practice observing any judgmental thoughts with the conveyor belt exercise from Exercise 1, remembering to wave at your judgments.

In the space below, briefly write about your practice of adopting a non-judgmental stance throughout this next week.

_____

_____

_____

_____

_____

_____

❑ I have practiced adopting a nonjudgmental stance this week.

❑ I have practiced the conveyor belt exercise (Exercise 1) at least twice this week.

HOMEWORK EXERCISE 6-B

Practicing Focusing on One Thing in the Moment

Practice focusing on one thing in the moment during the activities of your everyday life. For example, practice focusing on one thing in the moment while brushing your teeth, combing your hair, folding laundry, cooking, or listening to music. Try it for 30 seconds and gradually build up. This is something that you can practice every day. In the space below, briefly describe the activities during which you practiced this skill. What was it like? Were there any times that practicing focusing on one thing in the moment interrupted the chain that led to binge eating?

_____

_____

_____

_____

_____

_____

❑ I have practiced using focusing on one thing in the moment every day this week.

HOMEWORK EXERCISE 6-C

Practicing Being Effective with a Current Situation

Think of a situation in your current life where your focus on what is fair or how you would like things to be different is leading to urges to binge and interfering with your ability to identify what is really important to you. How can you practice the skill of being effective, keeping your focus on your goals and the actions you need to take to achieve them?

_____

_____

_____

_____

_____

❑ I have practiced being effective with a current situation.

❑ I have filled out my Diary Card daily.

❑ I have filled out at least one Behavioral Chain Analysis Form this week, either on a past binge or right when I was experiencing an urge to binge, or even just thinking about binge eating. (Note: At this point in the program, if you have not done so already, we encourage you to find out whether the act of filling out the Behavioral Chain Analysis Form and identifying skills you could use to break the chain is enough to prevent urges to binge from turning into binges or to allow you to cut off binges at their early stages. As you gain skill in being mindful, you may find yourself actually becoming able to "wake up" and become aware that, in that very moment, you are living a link on your chain. This can allow you to mentally recognize you are at Step 4 and substitute a skill as part of Step 5, effectively breaking your chain in real time.)

❑ I have used the skills I find most helpful so that I can use my wise mind and keep urges from turning into binges or cut off binges at their early stages.

7

Staying on Track

You have now worked through approximately half of this program. We've introduced you to new ideas and asked you to make a number of changes. You were taught new skills to increase your ability to cope more effectively with your emotions so that you can ultimately stop binge eating.

In this chapter you have the opportunity to review your progress to date. This review is important at the halfway point so you can reflect on how things have been going *and* where you may still need work (a dialectic between accepting where you are and asking yourself to work toward where you want to be). You may discover, for instance, that your binge eating has been decreasing but that you haven't been putting as much effort into the program lately and your motivation needs a boost. Or perhaps you're not seeing the improvements you had hoped for and you need help figuring out what is not working and what changes to make going forward.

This review focuses on the first two steps toward getting the life you want that we introduced in Chapter 3: stopping any behaviors that interfere with using this program and stopping binge eating. Please have all of your completed Diary Cards and Behavioral Chain Analysis Forms available for reference.

Step 1: Stop Any Behaviors That Interfere with Using This Program

As stated in Chapter 3, this program can work for you only if you're actively engaged—reading the chapters, completing the assigned exercises and homework, and using the Diary Card and Behavioral Chain Analysis Forms to record and analyze how to apply your new skills. So we asked you to watch out for interfering behaviors throughout the program. Now we ask you to assess whether any behaviors could be getting in the way of your being actively engaged with this program:

1. Have you been able to complete the chapters at the generally recommended speed (one chapter every week or two—we know some of these chapters are long!) while completing the associated exercises? If not, think about the primary factors that have interfered. Describe them below.

   _____

   _____

   _____

   _____

   _____

   _____

2. Have you been completing the homework after each chapter? If not, think about the primary factors that have interfered. Describe these below.

   _____

   _____

   _____

   _____

   _____

3. Have you been filling out your Diary Card each day? If not, think about the primary factors that have interfered. Describe these below.

   _____

   _____

   _____

   _____

   _____

   _____

4. Have you been filling out a Behavioral Chain Analysis Form at least once a week? If not, please think about the primary factors that have interfered. Describe these below.

_____

_____

_____

_____

_____

_____

If you answered yes to each of the four questions above, you can skip to "Step 2: Stop Binge Eating," on page 131. If you responded no to any of them, this is the time to think about how to manage the primary factors that interfered so you can get the maximum benefit from this program.

When John reviewed his progress, he noted that during the past 2 weeks he had not filled out a Diary Card every day and had not filled out any Behavioral Chain Analysis Forms. He had stopped binge eating for a number of weeks but had had some small binges these past 2 weeks. He was upset at himself for not making the program more of a priority and felt he would have completely stopped binge eating by now if he had.

John had found the skills of observing, adopting a nonjudgmental stance, and being effective helpful when he had tried to use them to reduce his binge eating, but he told us he was having difficulty applying these skills. To adopt a nonjudgmental stance, he thought about how he would approach a good friend in a similar situation, someone he would treat kindly and not automatically jump to criticize as he did himself. This was a strategy that he had found helpful before. With a good friend, he would begin by just observing the facts and without judging his friend as morally good or bad. Looking at his own case, the facts themselves were that he was spending less time on his Diary Cards and on filling out the Behavioral Chain Analysis Forms. It was also a fact that over the past couple of weeks the demands of his job had been greater. The consequences he noticed were that he was not thinking about the skills as often and his urges to binge were higher overall.

Instead of wasting energy criticizing himself, he tried to focus on being effective. What did he need to change to see a decrease in his binge eating and to more consistently fill out his Diary Cards and Behavioral Chain

Analysis Forms? The answer, he felt, was that he needed to prioritize the program so that he had fewer demands on his time. One option was to move some of his work commitments to later in the year, which would allow him more time now for working on the program. His wise mind accepted that there simply wasn't enough time to devote to everything he wanted to accomplish. Perhaps he might even explain to his boss that he needed some extra time to work on some health-related goals. His wise mind reminded him that before he started this program he had been binge eating almost every evening and had felt miserable much of the time. He took the opportunity to give himself credit for the progress he had made in the program. Using dialectical thinking, he accepted himself and his binge eating as it was now and decided to recommit to the program and change his behaviors from this point forward, beginning with filling out a Diary Card for that day. He also decided he would speak to his boss tomorrow.

EXERCISE 1 Strategies to Overcome Factors That Interfere with Your Using This Program

Go ahead now and write your strategy to overcome the obstacles that are getting in the way of your using this program to its full potential. If you answered yes to some of the questions but no to others, it might be useful to reflect on what has helped you follow through on these *yes* responses. Would any of those strategies be helpful for areas in which you are having trouble working through the program?

_____

_____

_____

_____

_____

_____

_____

_____

_____

_____

_____

Kat wrote:

I identified that I was not keeping up with reading a chapter every week or two because I was "too busy" and simply didn't have the time to spend.

I did a behavioral chain analysis and tried to use the skills of observing, being nonjudgmental, focusing on one thing in the moment, and being effective. My problem behavior was not keeping up with the weekly pace of reading the chapters and completing the exercises. My vulnerability had to do with my motivation. When I started this program, I felt determined to do whatever it would take to stop binge eating and live up to my potential. But because I started to stop binge eating, I felt like I was doing well, that the program was working, and so I felt less urgency to do the work as quickly and completely. Other priorities have taken over.

My plan to address this is to look over my exercises in Chapter 2 to remind myself why I committed to this program. I will review my values and what I imagined while gazing into a crystal ball and what I imagined my life would look like after I stopped binge eating.

After this, I felt motivated to look at a few things in my schedule I could change, at least for a while, to give me more time to read the chapters on time. I understand that even though I had stopped binge eating, I still needed to continue doing all the reading and homework to increase my chances of remaining free of binge eating no matter what life might throw at me.

The exercises and homework expose you to all the skills, at least once—and you never know which ones might truly become most effective for you. Just reading about the skills is not the same as actually attempting to use them, of course, so we recommend going back and completing any exercises and homework that you have not yet done.

Step 2: Stop Binge Eating

Take a moment and reflect on how you've been doing with stopping binge eating. Think about what has been working and what hasn't. Begin with looking back at how often each week you have binged since starting treatment.

Review your Diary Cards from the very start of the program and count how many binge episodes you had during each week. Try to remember roughly how many binge episodes you had the week before you started the program.

We know that you may not be sure of exactly what "counts" as a binge. As we described earlier, binges are commonly defined as episodes in which you experience a loss of control. If the amount of food eaten during the episode was excessive compared to what others would eat during that period and you felt you had lost control, we suggest that you label it as a large binge. If the amount was not excessive, but you experienced a loss of control, label it as a small one.

For each week, list the total number of large binges you had (although you may wish to count both large and small binges). If there were days when you did not fill out your Diary Card, just use your best guess. Also, note that we've added spaces for extra weeks in case you've spent more than one week on each chapter.

EXERCISE 2 Plotting Binge Episodes over Time

Week 0 (week before you started this program) _____

Week 1 _____   Week _____

Week 2 _____   Week _____

Week 3 _____   Week _____

Week 4 _____   Week _____

Week 5 _____   Week _____

Week 6 _____   Week _____

Week 7 _____   Week _____

Kat wrote:

Week 0 (week before you started this program) __7__

Week 1 __5__   Week 8 __1__

Week 2 __3__   Week 9 __2__

Week 3 __0__   Week _____

Week 4 __0__   Week _____

Week 5 __0__   Week _____

Week 6 __0__   Week _____

Week 7 __1__   Week _____

Sometimes it can be helpful to have a visual representation of behavioral changes you're making. If this is true for you, we suggest that you graph these numbers. We provide a sample graph on the facing page (top), followed by Kat's filled-in example (bottom).

On the vertical axis, write the numbers from 0 up to the highest number of binge-eating episodes a week you've had since beginning this program

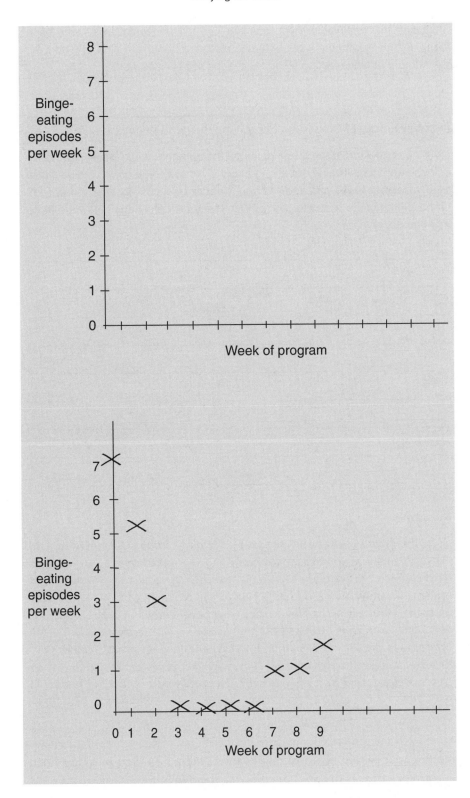

(including the week before you started). On the horizontal axis, write each week beginning with the week before you started treatment. Now plot an X for the number of binge-eating episodes that occurred each week.

EXERCISE 3 Describing Your Binge Eating Trend over Time

Now, either looking at the graph or just at the numbers you have written down, ask yourself the following questions about any trends you observe: Has there been a decrease? An increase? A choppy pattern of increases and decreases? Or have the numbers stayed pretty much the same? Describe below the trend that you observe.

_____

_____

_____

_____

_____

_____

_____

_____

_____

Kat wrote:

Over the first weeks of this program, my binge eating decreased pretty rapidly. I was having large binges every day the week before I started, and by the time I was reading Chapter 2 (week 3 or so of the program) and made my commitment, I pretty much stopped binge eating. I was highly motivated and felt great and continued with no binges till about week 6. It was about then that I stopped reading as regularly. It took me a long time to get through Chapter 6, maybe 3 weeks, and I wasn't practicing the skills as often. I started binge eating again, with one binge per week, and then this last week I had two. It's week 9 of the program and I'm in Chapter 7.

Now is the time to put on your DBT coach hat to figure out what has been affecting your pattern of binge episodes over time. This means adopting a non-judgmental stance as you practice observing the trends in your binge eating and, while practicing being effective, deciding on a plan of action. We have given you some specific suggestions (in the sections below) depending on whether you have noticed an overall decrease in your binge eating since starting the program (the first section) or not (the second section). Read the section that best represents your general trend. Although you have not yet been taught the entire program, it is important to look at your progress thus far. Research has shown that when people are able to make changes early in treatment they tend to benefit more.

Decrease in Binge Eating over Time

IF YOU HAVE DRAMATICALLY REDUCED YOUR BINGE EATING

For those whose binge eating has been dramatically reduced at this point in the program, your efforts have made a difference! However, sometimes people cut back on their effort once they notice they're in less distress. We caution you against doing this because decreasing your effort before you have learned all the skills could result in a later return of your binge eating. It's similar to being prescribed an antibiotic for an infection. Even if your symptoms improve quickly, it's important to take the full prescribed course. Stopping abruptly can cause the bacteria to develop resistance, and your infection may return and be even more difficult to control. The positive longer-term results found in our research on this program have been based on individuals who tended to complete the entire program. The feedback that we got from these participants was that many of the most helpful skills they learned were taught in the last chapters. And remember, the skills build on the ones that come before them. Therefore, even if you're no longer binge eating, or you're binge eating far less than you were when you started, we urge you to continue so that you have the chance to learn every skill. Keep up the effort you've been making thus far. This effort will pay off. The skills *do* become second nature with practice and will not require as much of your time or attention.

Although we recommend that you keep reading, if you're not binge eating or feeling urges to do so, you can skip to the next section, on behavioral chain analysis (see page 143).

IF YOU HAVE DECREASED YOUR BINGE EATING SOMEWHAT BUT ARE STILL HAVING SOME BINGE-EATING EPISODES

It probably won't come as a surprise to you that the way to decrease your binge eating even more is to either do more of what has worked for you so far or add new skills or new ways of applying existing skills. Ideally, you combine the two strategies.

To do more of what has been effective for you, review your Diary Cards and the homework sections from each chapter. Which skills do you tend to circle most often? How often are you filling out your Diary Card? Then come up with a plan to increase your use of these skills.

EXERCISE 4 Plan to Increase Using Skills That Are Already Working

Use the space below to describe how you will **increase use of skills that have been working for you.**

_____

_____

_____

_____

_____

_____

_____

_____

_____

_____

Kat wrote:

Looking at my Diary Card, the skills that I need to use more often that are already working for me are wise mind, adopting a nonjudgmental stance, and diaphragmatic breathing. My plan to help me use these skills more is to start the morning renewing my commitment by going over my 3" x 5" card of the pros and cons of stopping binge eating. Then I will look at the back of my Diary Card, where I will highlight the skills I have learned and plan to fit in that day. I will carry my Diary Card in my purse so that when I practice my skill, I can immediately circle it. If I practice more than once, I can double- or triple-circle with different-colored pens (which is fun for me to do and will make things look colorful).

For the second strategy, please read the next section.

Binge Eating Has Increased or Stayed the Same over Time

This section is for people who are seeing an increase in their binge eating or have noticed no real change in how often they are bingeing. As you know, there are many possible factors related to binge eating. If your binge eating has not decreased by this point in the program, our first suggestion is to reflect on the strength of your commitment to stop binge eating. Take a moment to practice adopting a nonjudgmental stance while reflecting on how important your commitment is. If you still feel you are 100% committed to stopping binge eating and turning to the program first, continue reading. If you feel your commitment is not strong or you're unsure, we suggest that before continuing, you review Chapter 2. For example, reread your responses, making sure you completed all the exercises (or perhaps even redoing them) to help you strengthen this fundamental commitment.

The DBT emotion regulation model of binge eating introduced in Chapter 1 can provide a useful structure for addressing the reasons your binge eating has not decreased. In particular, look at the role of triggers or prompting events and how effectively you are able to use skills to cope with uncomfortable emotions.

EXERCISE 5 The Role of Triggering/Prompting Events When Your Binge Eating Has Increased or Not Changed

a. **Most common prompting events that led to a binge.** Look at Section 1 of the Behavioral Chain Analysis Forms you've completed thus far, where you described the prompting events. When those behavioral chain analyses ended in a binge, what were the most common triggers or prompting events you experienced? List them in the space below.

_____

_____

_____

_____

_____

_____

_____

_____

Kat wrote:

The most common prompting events from my chains that have led me to binge have been:

1. When my husband is in a bad mood and withdraws from me

2. When my husband brings home food from work

3. When I am cleaning up after guests have left a dinner party we hosted

4. After I've received criticism about my singing performance

b. **Identifying controllable triggers.** Take a few minutes to look over the triggers you listed. **Which of these triggers do you think you could have had control over or could have control over now?** Examples of potentially controllable triggering events that commonly lead to binge eating include having to put away tempting leftovers after a party, being alone for unstructured periods of time in your home, and having arguments with a spouse or housemate over household chores. Describe the potentially controllable triggers in the space below.

_____

_____

_____

Kat wrote:

My controllable triggers are my husband bringing home food from work and cleaning up after my guests leave a dinner party we've hosted.

c. **Reducing the likelihood of encountering triggers/prompting events.** For the triggers/prompting events you listed, think of ways to reduce the likelihood of encountering them. Describe the plans you come up with to control or reduce your most common triggers in the space below.

_____

_____

_____

_____

_____

_____

_____

_____

_____

Kat wrote:

1. I plan to approach my husband and tell him how triggering it is for me to have the food his clients give to him in the house. I will ask him if he would consider not bringing it home. Because I know he hates to waste food, I'll give him information about local food pantries close to his office where he can easily drop it off. I will also let him know how much I appreciate his help and how I believe this will make me feel better about myself.

2. I plan to package leftovers from dinner parties and give them to my guests on their way out. Will ask my husband to stay with me in the kitchen or even help while I am cleaning up, as I am less likely to binge if he is there. If he is not home or is not available, I will wrap the food up and put it in my car trunk to donate.

d. **Identifying triggers that you cannot control or reduce.** Of the triggers you listed above in **a,** identify those you feel you cannot control or reduce. This is not to say that it is inevitable you will binge in response to triggers you now feel to be outside of your control. The option to not binge eat is always there. It can be useful, however, to recognize common triggers that *appear* to be outside of your control so that you can decide to accept them, at least in the current moment. Which triggers or events seem to be outside of your control right now?

_____

_____

_____

_____

_____

Kat wrote:

When my husband is in a bad mood and withdraws or when someone criticizes my performance, I can remind myself that I do not have control over others' thoughts, feelings, or actions and that I don't have to punish myself.

Much of your response to an uncontrollable prompting event depends on how you react or cope with the uncomfortable emotions that it triggered, which brings us to the next section.

Using Skills to Cope More Effectively
with Uncomfortable Emotions

If your binge eating has not decreased (or if it has but you want an even greater reduction), you can increase the effectiveness of this program by making sure that you are fully making use of all the skills you've learned so far. There may be skills you are not using, or not using as often as you should, that could really make a difference in helping you change how you respond to intense emotions and/or enable you to reduce your vulnerability to experiencing them.

Look over your Behavioral Chain Analysis Forms and your Diary Cards. Below, we briefly list and give a short description of the skills taught so far in this program. As you compare the skills you have circled with the skills listed below, check or circle the skills you are not using on a regular basis (e.g., at least three times a week). If the short description below feels insufficient, please review the skill by referring to the pages mentioned.

We will be teaching you some valuable new skills in the coming chapters, but these existing skills provide a very useful foundation.

❑ **Renewing your commitment (Chapter 2):** This skill involves renewing as often as possible the formal commitment to stop binge eating that you made in Chapter 2. Are you beginning your day by rereading the cards you made of the pros of stopping binge eating and the cons of continuing to binge eat?

❑ **Wise mind (Chapter 3):** This skill involves getting in touch with a very deep and centered part of yourself in which your emotions and your rational responses are integrated. In wise mind, you are operating from your best self, and your decisions and actions are in line with your values. Do you practice accessing your wise mind as often as possible to break links that might lead to binge eating?

❑ **Diaphragmatic breathing (Chapter 3):** The skill of diaphragmatic breathing involves practicing deep breathing and focusing on your breath. This type of breathing lowers stress and can facilitate mindfulness, or your awareness of being "here and now" in the present moment. Are you practicing diaphragmatic breathing when you are experiencing the urge to binge eat, a preoccupation with food, emotional discomfort, and/or physical tension?

❑ **Dialectical thinking (Chapter 5):** The skill of dialectical thinking involves being able to think flexibly instead of getting stuck in emotion mind and its rigid, perfectionistic, "black-or-white" mindset. Are you practicing using dialectical thinking and the Olympic athlete metaphor so that you don't have to abandon your important goal of stopping binge eating, despite not always achieving it? Are you also thinking dialectically to help you accept conflicting feelings about giving up binge eating as well as accepting yourself exactly as you are right now *and* committing to change?

❑ **Observing (Chapter 5):** This skill offers you the opportunity to experience physical sensations as well as intense emotions without getting caught up in, judging, or reacting to them. Are you practicing observing to help you become unstuck from your emotion mind and make it easier to access your wise mind?

These next three skills help you practice observing more skillfully.

❑ **Adopting a nonjudgmental stance (Chapter 6):** This skill involves not judging yourself or your emotions or behaviors in moral terms—such as good or bad, right or wrong, worthwhile or worthless. Are you practicing adopting a nonjudgmental stance toward yourself? For example, instead of making judgmental self-statements like "I'm a failure" or "I shouldn't be feeling this way—I'm a terrible person," are you practicing observing just the facts, remembering that you can accept how you feel without necessarily approving of it or acting on it? Are you adopting a nonjudgmental stance to help you move from emotion mind to wise mind to avoid binge eating?

❑ **Focusing on one thing in the moment (Chapter 6):** This skill involves not multitasking but, instead, placing your entire focus or attention on one thing, for one moment at a time. Are you practicing focusing on one thing in the moment on a regular basis to help you direct your attention, without letting your mind wander to something else? Have you been getting the most you can from this skill by taking opportunities to give yourself a break and slow down so that you can access your wise mind to help you deal with urges to binge eat?

❑ **Being effective (Chapter 6):** This skill means giving up being right, correct, or perfect, and/or the view that things must be exactly as you want them to be. Instead, acting effectively means doing what is needed to reach your goals. In some cases you *may* be right and your way *may* be the fair way, but being effective requires accepting the realities of the situation you are in during that moment. Are you practicing being effective to stop binge eating and get the most out of this program?

If you have not been using some of the skills listed above, it is important to make sure you start practicing them.

Take a moment and list the skills you are going to use more frequently:

_____

_____

_____

_____

_____

_____

Kat wrote:

1. Focusing on one thing in the moment

2. Being effective

3. Dialectical thinking

What if you feel that your binge eating occurs so quickly that it seems you are not aware of what is going on inside of you in time for you to realize you need to use a skill? Some of our patients describe feeling like this, especially in the first half of the program.

Look over your list of prompting events from your Behavioral Chain Analysis Forms that led you to binge eat (see Exercise 5, item a, on page 137). Familiarize yourself with this list of prompting events so that as soon as one occurs you become aware of it and can begin utilizing a skill in response. For example, if you find that getting into an argument with friends or family members is a trigger for you, begin using the skills as soon as you're aware that you are raising your voice or others are raising theirs. The skill of observing is especially valuable to help increase your awareness of the current situation. For example, as soon as you observe a feeling of tightness in your chest, you could immediately begin diaphragmatic breathing. It's good practice to use a skill whenever a prompting event takes place, even if it turns out that it might not be necessary and you are not likely to binge.

Below, list your most common trigger (from your list in Exercise 5 or additional ones you have thought of). List the earliest external and internal events you will practice observing in relation to the trigger (e.g., voice raised, fist clenched, sound of television turned on, freezer door opening), and list the skill(s) you will use as quickly as possibly once any of these occur:

_____

_____

_____

_____

_____

_____

_____

_____

_____

Kat wrote:

My most common trigger is when my husband comes home and isn't communicating with me. Looking at my Behavioral Chain Analysis Forms or even thinking about it now, I can see that one of the earliest signs is the tone in his voice when he says hello to me in a way that shows he doesn't want to talk to me. That tone triggers my self-blame. I tell myself that he isn't attracted to me, I'm too old, etc. The minute I hear that tone in his voice I will try to adopt a nonjudgmental stance and remind myself of all the other reasons that could be why he isn't communicating.

Behavioral Chain Analysis

We ask that you read this section regardless of what changes you have made in your binge eating so far. For example, even if you have stopped binge eating completely, you can use behavioral chain analysis to work on decreasing some other behavior from Step 3 or 4 of the program goals in Chapter 3 to get the life you want: mindless eating, involvement in apparently irrelevant behaviors, and compulsive shopping, for example. Perhaps your binge eating is commonly triggered by getting into arguments with others. Once you are no longer binge eating even when getting into arguments, you can use this program to work on not getting into unproductive arguments.

The behavioral chain analysis can be used in two main ways: (1) to analyze what happened and (2) to analyze what is happening *as it is occurring.*

After a binge-eating episode, the behavioral chain analysis allows you to adopt a nonjudgmental stance and examine what led to binge eating as well as to come up with strategies to prevent these triggers from happening again. Also, if you sense you are on the path toward a binge, immediately beginning a behavioral chain analysis will you give time to slow down and think about the different skills you could be using.

Review your Behavioral Chain Analysis Forms. Describe an example of when you used this powerful tool to analyze a binge that took place and analyze a binge (or urge to binge) *as it was occurring*. If you did not have examples of one or the other, write down your plan to use the chain in the way you did not use it during this coming week.

Kat wrote:

I notice that in the past 3 weeks or so I did not use the behavioral chain analysis in the moment to deal with an urge to binge. I also realize that I no longer am carrying around blank chains with me during the day. The two are probably related! I plan to print out five blank Behavioral Chain Analysis Forms and carry them in my purse (along with my Diary Card) so I will always have immediate access to them.

Maximizing Your Benefit from This Program

We hope this review was helpful and that you feel more aware of what is working and what isn't as we move forward and discuss more skills and strategies. If you can think of strategies we missed that would be helpful to you, use them as well.

This chapter focused on the first two steps to get the life you want. If you've been able to reach the first two steps and have stopped binge eating, you should be trying to reach Steps 3 and 4, which addresses other eating and noneating problem behaviors. You will find that the skills you have already begun to learn, such as the behavioral chain analysis, can easily be applied to other problem behaviors. You may find it helpful to refer to Chapter 3 to remind yourself of the different problem behaviors that were discussed.

Chapter 7 Summary

The purpose of this chapter was to help you take some time to reflect on your progress up to this point in the program. We hope that as you worked through this chapter you were able to adopt a nonjudgmental stance while observing the information you reviewed. We gave you specific recommendations based on whether you have had difficulty sticking with the program's assignments and/or difficulty in reducing your binge eating. As part of these recommendations, we reviewed some of the major skills we taught you so far to help you regulate emotions and thus decrease your binge eating. We also reviewed the behavioral chain analysis and asked you to reflect on how useful you found this tool. Finally, we asked you to think about whether there were any other activities you could be practicing to stop binge eating.

Homework

HOMEWORK EXERCISE 7-A
Taking the Opportunity to Review Skills/Concepts
from Earlier Chapters

If after working on this chapter you think there are any skills or concepts you need to review, please go back to the appropriate chapters and review them.

❑ I have read the relevant chapter(s) for the skills or ideas I needed to review.

❑ I have filled out my Diary Card daily.

❑ I have filled out at least one Behavioral Chain Analysis Form this week.

❑ I have used the skills I find most helpful so that I can access my wise mind to stop binge eating before it starts.

8

Mindful Eating and Urge Surfing

We hope the review in the last chapter was helpful. We're now going to turn our attention back to mindfulness. Mindfulness—being able to nonjudgmentally accept yourself and the situation you are in—is the foundation you need to manage your emotions without turning to binge eating. That's because mindfulness and binge eating are completely incompatible. Mindfulness is about increasing your awareness, whereas binge eating is about shutting down your awareness. By definition, binge eating is mind*less*. You cannot practice mindfulness and at the same time binge eat, just as your body cannot be simultaneously tense and relaxed. To binge eat, you cannot be mindful.

Mindful Eating

Mindful eating is a way to focus your attention on what you are eating and allows you to listen to your body and better tell when you are hungry or full. This requires applying three mindfulness skills to the activity of eating: observing, adopting a nonjudgmental stance, and focusing on one thing in the moment. When you practice mindful eating, you eat each bite of food with full awareness, consciousness, and attention to each moment, each taste, each chew.

But that's not all you're aware of. Leticia explained how many of her binge-eating episodes involved her feeling fully awake to the tastes, flavors, and sensations of the different foods she ate, so she thought she was being mindful and binge eating at the same time. She felt like she was paying attention and was fully in the moment. We pointed out, however, that while Leticia was fully aware of the tastes of the food, she was *not* fully aware of her core values and deep commitment to her long-term best interests. In this very important sense, she was shutting out of her awareness the realities of what she was doing.

After thinking about these points, Leticia became aware that after a binge she often felt as if she was emerging from a "fog." She deeply regretted her actions and never could quite believe that she had allowed herself to lose sight of her goals.

Like Leticia, you may feel that you are fully in the moment when you binge. However, we think you would agree that some part of you is choosing to shut down your awareness of the consequences you will eventually face. When you are bingeing, a core part of you is on autopilot. Your wise mind—the part of you in touch with your core values and the quality of life you hope to have—is not accessible.

EXERCISE 1 Can a Binge Be Mindful?

How does defining binge eating as mindless fit your experience? Do you think it's possible to binge and also listen to your wise mind, or do you feel part of you is choosing to shut down awareness of the longer-term consequences of your behavior? Have you ever had a binge that, afterwards, left you feeling whole and good about yourself, a binge that you didn't ultimately regret?

Write your answer in the space below.

_____

_____

_____

_____

_____

_____

_____

Kat wrote:

I thought maybe a binge can be mindful, as sometimes I felt that I make a choice to binge because there is no other option. But when I really thought about it, I realized that I am using binge eating to avoid feeling and that I am not in control. I swallow my food in big gulps quickly, and I am not enjoying the experience of eating or even being present. I realize that there is no way that binge eating is compatible with mindfulness.

Most patients we have worked with either initially or eventually agree that binge eating *is* mindless eating. Mindful eating, on the other hand, is about being able to slow down and eat with full awareness as you stay in touch with your core values and deep commitment to your long-term best interests.

EXERCISE 2   Experiencing Mindful Eating

First, choose a food to practice on. We suggest raisins to start with since they are a food that many people tend to eat by the handful, without ever having eaten just one. However, you can practice mindful eating with any food. If you find raisins too tempting, choose a small portion of a less tempting food (e.g., a small piece of broccoli, a cup of tea). If all foods seem too tempting outside of a planned meal, you can practice mindful eating with a food during a planned meal or snack. It is also helpful to first practice mindful eating when you are not experiencing strong emotions or are otherwise feeling triggered to binge eat. Use your wise mind. What is important is having the opportunity to experience what it means to eat with full awareness.

"Take three raisins and hold them in your hand. Begin by observing the raisins in your palm, bringing your attention to each one.

"Observe each raisin carefully. You might imagine that you're a Martian, seeing a raisin for the first time. Really observe. For example, notice the different shapes, surfaces, and colors. Notice the texture with your fingertips. While you are observing, be aware of any thoughts that come into your mind about raisins or eating raisins before gently setting the raisins down.

"Now bring just one raisin to your nose and smell it. Fully immerse yourself in the smell of one raisin. Then, with awareness of your arm and hand moving, place the raisin in your mouth. Be aware of your mouth, your tongue. Then experience the taste of one raisin by chewing it very slowly. Notice the texture on your tongue, on the roof of your mouth. Notice how the raisin feels as you bite into it with your teeth. Notice any impulses to swallow the raisin. Then, when you are ready, swallow it—following the

---

About This Exercise

The original version of this exercise appeared in *Full Catastrophe Living* by Jon Kabat-Zinn, who has used mindfulness as a basis for a stress-reduction program he started at the University of Massachusetts Medical Center. These mindfulness skills were found to be effective for reducing pain in individuals suffering from chronic pain syndromes. Our version has been greatly modified.

taste as long as you can as it goes down your throat. Fully observe the experience of eating just this one raisin.

"Eat each of the three raisins in this way, chewing each one slowly, really tasting, noticing where the raisin is in your mouth, listening to the sounds of the chewing, being fully aware. . . . Notice whether there are any differences between the first raisin and the others. Does the taste change now that you've already eaten one? Notice your experience with each chew. You are mindfully eating—putting all your attention and awareness on this one thing you are doing. You are literally more awake—the opposite of mechanically eating. You are focusing your full attention on eating."

Write about what that mindful eating exercise was like for you in the space below. You may wish to read about John's experience with mindful eating in the box on page 150.

_____

_____

_____

_____

_____

_____

_____

_____

_____

_____

Kat wrote:

This was a powerful exercise for me. I immediately noticed that the minute I smelled the sweetness of the raisin I had an overwhelming urge to shove it in my mouth and swallow it. I even found myself looking around for the next thing to put into my mouth. By slowing down, and forcing myself to wait, I noticed things about the raisin I never had before. That the wrinkles looked like fingerprints. When I finally tasted the raisin, slowly examining it, I found the sweetness was almost too much, and when I really paid attention, I found that I didn't want any more. It was amazing to me that I could not want to eat more of something so sweet.

John's Experience with Mindful Eating

Like many of our patients, John identified eating mindlessly as a big trigger for him. The binge he described in Chapter 1 involved eating ice cream while watching TV. "Sometimes I won't even be aware of how much I've eaten till I notice how much of the container is gone. And then I feel so angry at myself that I figure I might as well finish off the whole thing!" Not only did he come to realize he ate mindlessly, but his parents had never paid much attention to mealtimes. The family rarely sat down at the table, but tended to eat while watching TV or while talking on the phone. Turning off the TV and practicing mindful eating with nonbinge foods allowed John to slow down and start tasting and appreciating the food he ate every day. As he became more comfortable, he decided to practice mindful eating with small portions of ice cream. He noticed that practicing mindful eating enabled him to enjoy the ice cream much more and he was much more willing and able to stop once he had finished his portion.

Using Mindful Eating to Prevent a Binge

If you practiced mindful eating every time you ate, by definition, you would never binge. However, given how much time it takes to eat every bite of food with full awareness, we understand this would likely be impractical. How, then, can you use this skill to prevent binge eating?

One suggestion is that you practice mindful eating, initially with nontempting (e.g., nonbinge) foods so that you develop a body sense of what it feels like to eat this way—a "muscle memory." We explain the importance of this to our patients by describing how rehearsals for a play, although different from the actual performance, are necessary and useful. The adrenaline of having a live audience is missing, but having had frequent rehearsals allows you to move your body through the actual motions and to say the actual words that you will use during the real performance. Similarly, practicing mindful eating when you are not stressed is helpful for times when you are vulnerable to a binge and want to prevent one.

For example, say you are at a restaurant with friends or family. If the conversation becomes argumentative, you're likely to feel uncomfortable emotions that might lead you to overeat and then binge. However, if you've practiced mindful eating, you'll have a muscle memory that can help you stay present and aware. Although it would not be practical to mindfully eat your entire meal, you could mindfully eat a few bites and then participate in the conversation (without eating). Then you could mindfully take a few more bites. You won't be able to mindfully eat your entire meal, but you could eat the most tempting foods as mindfully as possible.

What mindful eating offers, especially when you're vulnerable to bingeing, is the opportunity to slow down and focus so that your awareness of what you're doing can "catch up" with your actual behaviors. Research shows that the feeling of fullness often requires at least 20 minutes to occur. Mindful eating allows your brain enough time to signal your stomach that your physical hunger has diminished. When you concentrate with full awareness on every bite of food, it's much easier to make contact with your wise mind and prevent a binge.

One question you may be asking is whether or not you should practice mindful eating with a binge food. Many patients we have worked with have been able to do this and have found that doing so helps them prevent a binge or stop a binge from progressing. The key is not to attempt to mindfully eat a binge food too soon. One of the ways to practice building up to it is with a technique called imaginal mindful eating. We explain how to use this in the following exercise. One advantage of learning how to mindfully eat binge foods is that engaging in black-and-white thinking about food (labeling some foods as "good" and others as "bad") can trigger a binge. We will discuss this more fully in Chapter 10, in the section on balancing your eating.

EXERCISE 3 Imaginal Mindful Eating

Note: We recommend practicing this exercise beginning with one of your less tempting binge foods and building your way up as you gain confidence. For example, if your favorite binge foods tend to be sweet rather than salty, you might start imagining yourself eating pretzels or chips before doing this exercise with foods you find more tempting, such as candy or sugary desserts.

"Begin by sitting on a chair. Let the chair fully support you, with your feet on the floor and your head aligned as if a string were attached from it to the ceiling. Find a place for your eyes to focus softly that won't distract you. Take several deep, flowing breaths and imagine a food that you might typically binge on.

"Then bring your full, undivided attention to just this food as you did with the raisins. Smell the food, look at it, observe its color. Take one chew at a time, experiencing one flavor at a time—with your full attention on the act of eating, on tasting, on chewing.

"You might be aware of thoughts or emotions. Notice them, but keep your attention on the activity of eating. If your mind wanders, gently bring it back to the activity you're engaged in, one small swallow at time."

What was your imaginal mindful eating like? Describe it in the space below.

_____

_____

_____

_____

_____

_____

Kat wrote:

After the experience with the raisin, I felt ready to practice on a tempting binge food. I chose to imagine mindfully eating a Yule log that my husband's client gives to him at the holidays. I have binged on this delicious treat for many years. I imagined cutting one slice, putting it on a plate, and observing it as if it I had never seen it before or had any experience with it. I smelled it. I enjoyed observing the smells and how it looked even before putting the tiniest bite in my mouth! By the time I imagined taking a bite, I was already feeling satisfied and calm and was able to see myself chewing slowly, enjoying the spongy softness. I don't know if I will ask my husband not to bring the Yule log this year, but I feel that if he does, it might be nice to enjoy it in just this way.

Unlike what most people might think, imaginal exercises usually don't increase a person's urge to binge. However, if you found that this exercise made you want to binge, this is a perfect opportunity to use all your skills to nonjudgmentally observe this urge and let it pass. In fact, the technique of observing the urge is called urge surfing and is the skill you're about to learn.

Urge Surfing

Urge surfing allows you to ride out your urges to binge eat, giving you time to access your wise mind and help you prevent an actual binge episode.

This skill involves using mental imagery—in this case, visualizing your urge to binge as if it were a wave on the ocean. Urge surfing involves learning to "surf" this wave, or "surf" your urges to binge eat. When you practice this skill, you use the mindfulness skills of observing, focusing on one thing in the moment, and adopting a nonjudgmental stance to stay with the experience of the urge without succumbing to it or intensifying it by judging it or yourself. By observing the ebb and flow of your urge, you are separating the urge from the object of the urge—the binge. By noticing your urges moment by moment, you are able to maintain awareness of how your urge, like a wave, evolves and shifts over time. Intense urges are time-limited and will end if you do not give in to them.

Urge surfing involves visualizing yourself with your feet actually on a surfboard, riding the crest of the wave. When you first notice an urge to binge and begin to urge surf, the urge or wave will likely seem quite large—just like an actual wave when a surfer first catches it. As you start to surf, you may sense that the urge keeps growing bigger and bigger. However, over time—as you continue to surf—you will notice that the urge fluctuates in strength, rising and falling. Instead of trying to control the wave's movement, urge surfing asks you to stay on top of the wave as it rises and falls, rises and falls . . . until you have ridden the urge fully out and are at the shore.

How Urge Surfing Works

Research shows that intense urges not only do not last forever, but typically last about 20 minutes. As you practice urge surfing, the duration of urges will decrease over time. Urge surfing works because it retrains your brain. In the past, every time you automatically gave in to an urge to binge, you reinforced the link between having an urge and acting on it.

When you detach yourself from your urges through urge surfing, your brain learns it is possible to experience an urge *without* acting on it. Gradually your brain's new knowledge weakens the old link between having an urge and acting on it. Every time you use your mindfulness skills of observing, adopting a nonjudgmental stance, and focusing on one thing in the moment to "surf" your urges to binge, you are taking advantage of a key opportunity to retrain your brain and unlearn old patterns.

EXERCISE 4 Practicing Urge Surfing

Choose something to practice urge surfing with. For your first experience, you should pick something of relatively low intensity. You may wish to practice with urges that do not involve food, such as your urges to check a text message, to purchase something online, or to keep watching a Netflix show instead of going to sleep. This is what Angela did (described on the next page).

The image of a wave is a useful metaphor for the experience of being caught up in any urge and noticing a strong pull to act in a way that is consistent with that urge. When you feel more comfortable with your ability to urge surf and are ready to practice with food, practice first with foods that you like but don't have cravings for. If all foods feel too tempting at first, practice urge surfing using your imagination. As you gain experience and confidence, you can build up to practicing with actual foods and then more and more tempting foods.

> "Begin by putting the food (or nonfood, if that is how you choose to start) in front of you. If it's a food, don't eat it. Simply observe it with your senses—looking, smelling, listening. Stay mindful of any thoughts, feelings, or judgments that may arise. Be very aware of any action urges, such as urges to eat the food, check the phone, website, etc. Do your best to be open to whatever comes to mind. Remind yourself that the idea is to stay present with the urges without acting on them. Experience yourself as a surfer, riding the wave of your urge as it rises and falls, rises and falls. As you surf the urge, watch the wave rise higher and higher and then start to fall. You may notice the belief that your urge will never stop rising, but practicing urge surfing will allow you to experience for yourself that the urge WILL always fall.
>
> "Use observing, adopting a nonjudgmental stance, and focusing on one thing in the moment with all that you experience—any thoughts, sensations, feelings, or judgments. Sometimes visualizing the tempting food as if it were a picture or photograph may be helpful in detaching yourself from it.
>
> "Continue to urge surf until you have ridden out the urge. It's OK if this takes some time."

At the end of this exercise, practice getting in touch with your wise mind to decide whether to act on the urge. If you choose to eat the food, check the texts, make the purchase, be sure you do so as a mindful, conscious choice. If you choose not to satisfy the urge, be mindful of that experience.

One very valuable benefit of urge surfing is that it gives you time to think about what's really going on, instead of just acting on your urges. This was particularly relevant for Angela.

Angela's first attempts at urge surfing didn't go very well. She would notice an intense urge to binge and try to just let it sit there. However, the urge seemed to get stronger and stronger until she would end up bingeing—so she gave up using urge surfing. When we discussed Angela's disappointing experiences with this skill, we suggested she back up and try it on fairly low-intensity urges that did not involve food so that she could regain confidence. She was skeptical but willing to try. For her, fairly low-intensity urges involved checking texts on her phone and looking at updates on Facebook while she was at work and continuing to read instead of going to sleep even when she was very tired. She was pleased to see that she really could have an urge and not have to act on it. Practicing urge surfing with these non-eating-related urges increased her sense of confidence. One day, arriving home after a long day that had included a difficult interaction with her boss, she experienced a sudden urge to binge that felt like it "hit" her "out of the blue." Angela decided she felt ready to practice urge surfing, but, to be safe, she stayed away from the kitchen and went upstairs to her bedroom. Sitting in a recliner chair, she practiced experiencing her urge to binge as a wave that kept rising and falling, coming and going, in the same way that her urges to check Facebook had come and gone. She reminded herself that she didn't need to be frightened of the urge, that having urges didn't mean having to act on them.

After only 15 minutes, Angela was surprised that she no longer experienced the urge to binge. The wave had receded. As she practiced diaphragmatic breathing, she found herself able to access her wise mind. She realized that her urge to binge was a distress signal. She had been feeling upset and drained from her day, and although at the time the urge had felt like it came out of the blue, she could now connect the dots and realize she wanted soothing. Taking the time to practice urge surfing felt like a huge success. She decided to relax on her recliner a bit longer and read a short magazine article to give herself more time for self-care. She then felt ready to have dinner with her family without struggling further with urges to binge eat for the rest of the evening.

Sometimes our patients are skeptical about whether or not urge surfing can actually work for them. The connection between having an urge and giving in to that urge is so familiar for most people who binge eat that they often can't separate the experience of the urge from the experience of capitulating to it. However, after you've practiced urge surfing several times, we're confident you will begin to see that giving in to an urge is a choice you can actively make or *not* make. It is not easy, especially at first, but we know from the many patients we have worked with who love urge surfing that you can do it!

EXERCISE 5 Planning Ways to Use Mindful Eating and/or Urge Surfing to Prevent a Binge

This chapter has offered you different exercises to practice mindful eating and urge surfing. Hopefully, you now have at least a sense for how these skills could work for you. This exercise asks you to think about the coming weeks and ways you can incorporate mindful eating and urge surfing to prevent bingeing. For example, suppose you have a social event on your schedule that involves food. Your plan might involve going to the event, choosing what you wish to eat, and then practicing mindful eating for several bites and carrying on a conversation when you're not eating. However, if you know that you tend to be vulnerable to overeating at social events, particularly if you're anxious about meeting new people, your plan might include urge surfing as soon as you become aware of any urges to binge. Or, if you begin overeating, are moving toward a binge, and are unwilling or unable to practice urge surfing, you might choose to return to mindful eating as a way to slow yourself down, access your wise mind, and then start urge surfing if the urges persist.

In the space below, write about your plans for practicing mindful eating and urge surfing in the coming weeks.

_____

_____

_____

_____

_____

_____

_____

Kat wrote:

I am having a few friends over for dinner, and my husband will be away. I know that when I am cleaning up I will have a huge urge to binge on the leftovers. Although I will try to package food for friends to take, there will no doubt be some food that remains. I will use urge surfing with the wave, watch it, and sit with it until it passes. I will then make a decision about whether to eat more of anything. If I do choose to eat any leftovers later that evening, I will practice mindful eating.

Chapter 8 Summary

This chapter introduced you to two new skills: mindful eating and urge surfing. Mindful eating involves bringing your full attention and awareness to the food you are eating. Binge eating is a mindless activity during which you shut out or deny full awareness of the consequences of your behavior. Mindful eating involves helping you access your wise mind when you are eating. When you practice mindful eating, you are using the skills of observing along with adopting a nonjudgmental stance and focusing on one thing in the moment.

The second skill discussed in this chapter was urge surfing. Urge surfing involves waiting for the urge to binge eat to decrease rather than giving in to it. As you urge surf, you use the skills of observing, adopting a nonjudgmental stance, and focusing on one thing in the moment to maintain awareness, moment by moment, of how your urge rises and falls and ultimately decreases.

We also discussed how both of these skills can play important roles in preventing binge eating. Mindful eating can decrease the chances that eating will turn into a binge, and urge surfing allows you to overcome the urge to have a binge-eating episode. Continued practice with these skills will give you much greater control of your relationship with food.

Homework

HOMEWORK EXERCISE 8-A
Mindful Eating Practice over the Coming Week

Plan to practice mindful eating at least once a day for the next week. Begin with foods that are relatively neutral before moving to more tempting foods. If all foods are too tempting, continue to practice imaginal eating. It can be helpful to choose different foods each time. Describe your experiences below.

Day 1: _____

_____

Day 2: _____

_____

Day 3: _____

_____

Day 4: _____

_____

Day 5: _____

_____

Day 6: _____

_____

Day 7: _____

_____

❏ I have practiced mindful eating once a day this week.

HOMEWORK EXERCISE 8-B

Urge Surfing Practice Over the Coming Week

Practice urge surfing at least three times this week. Depending on your confidence about using this skill (listen to yourself and consult your wise mind!), you might wish to begin by practicing with urges that do not involve food or that use food imaginally. You may also want to practice by delaying eating the foods you plan to eat—but surfing the urge instead of immediately allowing yourself to eat.

When practicing with actual foods, make sure your early practices involve nontempting foods first. Then practice with increasingly tempting foods (using imaginal food to gain confidence when needed). Write about your experience below.

_____

_____

_____

_____

_____

_____

_____

❑ I have practiced urge surfing at least three times this week.

❑ I have filled out my Diary Card daily.

❑ I have filled out at least one Behavioral Chain Analysis Form this week.

❑ I have used the skills I find most helpful so that I can use my wise mind and stop binge eating before it happens.

9

Being Mindful of Your Current Emotion and Radically Accepting Your Emotions

This chapter begins a new module, the *emotion regulation* skills. These skills will teach you to more directly manage distressing emotional states, decrease your vulnerability to painful emotions, and increase how often and how fully you experience positive emotions.

As we have discussed in previous chapters, the underlying assumption of this program is that individuals who binge eat experience emotional states they are ill equipped to manage skillfully. The emotion regulation skills will build on your mindfulness skills by extending your awareness and openness to the current moment so that it includes your full emotional experience.

We want to emphasize that the goal of the emotion regulation skills is *not* to eliminate negative or uncomfortable emotions. Distressing and difficult emotions are a part of life; they cannot be entirely avoided. However, what can be changed is the way you react to your distress and difficult emotions.

To help you respond to your emotions as skillfully as possible, it is valuable to be able to distinguish a *primary* emotion (the first, or original emotional reaction you have) from a *secondary* emotion (the emotion triggered by the primary emotion). For example, if you are afraid to speak to a group of people and instinctively feel fear, then fear is the primary emotion. If you attempt to block your fear by telling yourself to "snap out of it" and by calling yourself an "idiot," a secondary emotion is likely to be triggered, such as shame. Being able to name or label your primary emotion has been shown to decrease physiological arousal and activate centers in the brain related to greater control over behavior. On the other hand, attempts to block awareness of a primary emotion, or judge it as invalid or wrong, increase physiological arousal. Such attempts usually backfire because greater arousal potentially leads to greater urges to escape through turning to food.

Over 2,500 years ago, the Buddha recognized this problematic pattern of responding. He stated that we humans tend to cause ourselves unnecessary suffering by shooting ourselves with a "second arrow." Although the Buddha acknowledged that we cannot avoid all pain in life (getting shot with what he referred to as the "first arrow"), we can make wise choices and not cause ourselves additional suffering by following the first arrow with a second! All too often, individuals who binge eat shoot that second arrow by responding to their emotional pain with invalidating self-judgments.

Like many of our patients, you may have fallen into the trap of labeling your painful emotions as "the problem," rather than identifying the problem as your response to painful emotions—such as to turn to binge eating. Painful emotions, by definition, can be very distressing, but how you choose to act or not act on them is truly what is most critical. It is possible to respond to your primary painful feelings with understanding, interest, compassion, or countless other skillful reactions that may lead to a decrease in emotional intensity and an increased sense of mastery. We hope recognizing that your past relationship with your emotions was not always constructive will make you feel optimistic about the constructive changes you can make by adding the emotion regulation skills to the mindfulness skills from the previous chapters. Although in the short run binge eating may distract you from feeling certain emotions, it leads not only to a buildup of primary and secondary emotions, but also to devastating consequences that negatively affect your self-esteem, health, and general well-being.

Mindfulness of Your Current Emotion

Mindfulness of your current emotion will help you be fully aware of and open to the current moment, accepting all of your emotional experience and rejecting none of it. In using the mindfulness skills of observing, adopting a nonjudgmental stance, and focusing on one thing in the moment, you make an active choice to take a step back and separate yourself from your emotion so you can observe it with greater objectivity.

Often, when we have intense emotions, we tell ourselves we *are* our emotions (e.g., "I *am* sad" or "I *am* angry"). To make it easier to observe your emotion as separate from yourself you may wish, as do some of our patients, to create a visual image of your emotion. For example, you can think of your emotion as a river that is raging in front of you. If you were to jump into it, you would be swept away. However, by remembering that it is possible to pause and sit on the bank, you can watch the water rush by without being carried downstream by the rush of the river's strong feelings and into harm's way. You don't have to jump in. Instead, you can accept the river as you sit on the bank, observing your emotion as you adopt a nonjudgmental stance while focusing on one thing in the moment. Exercise 1 uses the image of your emotion as a crashing ocean wave.

Another way to use visualization is to picture your emotion as an object with its own particular size, shape, and color. One patient described her anger as an elephant-sized, fiery-red ball with sharp black spikes coming out in all directions. This object can be something outside your body, or you may find it helpful to practice observing your emotion within or on top of your body. For example, another patient described her guilt as a dark-colored, weighty mass circling and pressing down on her shoulders and upper chest. By using observing, focusing on one thing in the moment, and adopting a nonjudgmental stance, you can externalize and remain separate from your emotion while still being aware of it. The goal is not to attempt to suppress, block, or push your emotion away while also not attempting to hold on to, intensify, change, or "fix" it.

You can begin to get some experience with mindfulness of your current emotion by doing the following exercise. Some of our patients find it difficult to begin practicing with strong emotions and find it useful to begin with less intense emotions, as we describe below. Eventually, when you've built confidence in practicing this skill, you can use this exercise with more intense or overwhelming emotions.

EXERCISE 1 Practicing Mindfulness of Your Current Emotion

"Take a moment to sit in a chair, with your feet on the floor, your posture erect, while taking slow, easy breaths from your diaphragm. Find a place for your eyes to focus that does not distract you.

"Then bring to mind an emotional experience that you have been aware of recently. For the first few times that you practice this skill, choose an emotion that, while strong enough for you to be aware of it, is not intense or overwhelming. For instance, you may wish to practice by thinking of something in the news that does not directly affect you or those you love, such as having a reaction when you heard about the death of an admired musician, author, or actor; the cancellation of a television show you particularly enjoy; or hearing about the losing score for your favorite sports team. Once you've brought up and observed the emotion, see if you can identify what it was. Maybe you were saddened, mildly disappointed, surprised, annoyed, or anxious?

"Whatever the emotion is, try to imagine it as something separate or external from yourself such as a wave colliding with the shore only to be pulled back into the ocean as the process repeats. If you want to stay 'dry,' you will not try to block the wave. It would knock you over and could pull you out to sea. Instead, you practice focusing on one thing in the moment, staying with whatever is present, continuously bringing your attention back to the wave as you stand at the shore.

"Practice adopting a nonjudgmental stance by not judging the emotion or yourself for having it. Practice releasing or letting go of the emotional experience, reminding yourself that this experience isn't all of who you are and that inevitably all emotions shift and change. Practice fully accepting what is.

"Take several deep, flowing breaths and end the exercise."

Use the space below to describe what practicing mindfulness of your current emotion was like for you.

_____

_____

_____

_____

_____

_____

_____

_____

Kat wrote:

I found this difficult at first. I observed my right foot falling asleep, and I noticed the emotion of irritation. I wanted to get up and walk around but tried to observe my irritation like it was a wave. I tried to stay with that visual and found myself being judgmental that it was hard, which made me feel more irritable at first. When I realized this, I told myself "This is new, this is hard, it's OK—just focus on the wave." I was able to see myself as separate from my irritability and say, "This is not all of who I am. It will pass"—just like the exercise suggested. It was fascinating to see how the judgment made my feelings so much more intense.

As we described in Chapter 1, John was told as a child that it wasn't OK for him to cry, get angry, or in general to express his emotions. As an adult, before he started this program, he typically was unaware of having strong feelings. Over time, it became clearer to him that he actually did have strong emotions but had difficulty accessing them. It was as if he had an internal wall that he put up when he noticed his feelings becoming strong or intense. This made sense as he had had so little experience with his emotions that he did not trust his ability to cope with them without being overwhelmed. Instead, he had become accustomed to using negative self-judgments to invalidate his feelings and turning to mindless eating and binge eating to numb himself. It was only when the consequences of his eating behaviors became so distressing that he was willing to seek help. Like most of us, John found being mindful of his current emotion gave him a new option for approaching his emotions, although it took perseverance for him to learn to use the skill.

> John found the imagery of sitting alongside a bank observing his emotions as a river in front of him to be quite helpful. He wasn't always sure which of his emotions was primary or which was secondary, but he found that observing his emotions as separate from him helped him feel less responsible for controlling them. This made it easier for him to identify and label his emotions, which in and of itself was a powerful experience and helped him manage them more skillfully.
>
> After a frustrating business dinner at which he felt a supervisor was taking credit for work he had done, he came home feeling very distressed. Uncertain of exactly what he was feeling, he practiced being mindful of his current emotion as if it were a flowing river. As he sat on the bank and observed, he identified that he was feeling intense anger. He continued to observe and noticed that the anger was directed at himself: "Why are you so upset? This isn't such a big deal! Who cares if he took credit tonight—it's still your work. It will become clear eventually!" Noticing these self-judgments, he brought his attention back to observing the river. As he did so, he was surprised that he had become tearful and choked up. He identified that the emotion he was observing was sadness, and recognized that this was his primary emotion—one he had attempted to invalidate with the secondary emotion of anger. Externalizing his emotions as separate from himself enabled him to experience his sadness, which he wouldn't have recognized before, with depth and intensity. Practicing mindfulness of his current emotion, John was able to give himself permission to sit with his feelings without evoking the distressing emotional arousal that had played a major role in triggering his urges to binge in the past.

Radically Accepting Your Emotions

Fully accepting and being aware of your emotions can obviously be difficult, particularly if they are painful. That's likely why you turned to binge eating in the first place. *Radically accepting your emotions* is a skill that will help you tolerate emotions that you find difficult to experience and thus give you options other than binge eating.

The fact is that at times your life will involve situations you cannot change, or at least cannot change right away. *Radical acceptance* means accepting what you cannot change—while, of course, changing what you can. By accepting all of your emotional experiences, even the painful ones, you don't add "extra baggage" to your experience by fighting or resisting emotional discomfort through turning to food. *Suffering* can be defined as the struggle to keep pain out of your awareness and thus can be distinguished from pain itself. Struggling to escape or deny pain ensures that you remain engaged in the effort not to accept things as they are. While it is absolutely natural to want as little pain as possible, attempts to bury or avoid pain through binge eating or other attempts to block or escape pain ultimately add to the suffering that you experience. Being stuck fighting reality and not accepting pain generates and maintains suffering.

The good news is that the skill of radical acceptance can transform pain-plus-suffering into the simple experience of pain in this current moment. We can't overemphasize that radically accepting your emotions does not mean that your emotional pain goes away, and we are not suggesting that pain in this moment is easy to accept. This is why radically accepting your emotions is a skill that takes practice. The word *radical* is Latin for "root," and *radically* accepting your emotions involves accepting your feelings at their root or core—in a deep and fundamental way. Radically accepting your emotions is not a superficial acceptance of how you feel. Instead, it means accepting that painful emotions are part of the universal human experience and cannot be avoided. This is a reality that many of us have spent a lifetime trying to deny. Therefore, it's only natural that practice will be required to develop acceptance.

EXERCISE 2   Identifying the Emotion You Currently Find Hardest to Accept

We have noticed that our patients often have one emotion that is more difficult for them to accept than others. **Which emotion is currently the hardest for you to accept?** Write your response below.

_____

_____

_____

Kat wrote:

Anger is the most difficult emotion for me to accept. It feels terrifying because it makes me feel completely out of control. I worry that if I let myself express the rage I can feel, something terrible will happen.

A good way to think about radically accepting your emotion is to think about the principle behind the Chinese "finger puzzle." (If you are not familiar with it, read the description in the box below.)

The puzzle demonstrates how fighting to free your fingers ensures that they stay locked in the struggle, whereas letting go and ceasing to pull on your fingers releases them.

We want to stress that we understand how frightening and difficult it can be to let go of trying to control your feelings. But if you practice the skill of radically accepting your emotions, you *will* be able to focus your energy more productively. Think about having a leak in the oil pan of your car. One option in that situation is to avoid accepting the situation. In this case you'll waste time and energy checking the oil and complaining about how much money you're spending to replenish the oil. Staying engaged in this struggle distracts you from thinking about the larger issue, which requires accepting the existence of the leak and deciding what to do about it. While radically accepting the existence of the root problem rather than the symptom may not be pleasant, your chances of effectively addressing the problem are much greater. You still must address the pain of the situation, but you are not adding suffering.

Angela's husband had an affair several years before she started the program. She decided to stay with him. She told him that they should put it all behind them without ever acknowledging how angry and hurt she was. Whenever the thought of the affair popped into Angela's head, she pushed it away. In our work with her, Angela discovered that these thoughts preceded a fight with her husband and the urge to binge. Radically accepting her emotions required Angela to accept what had happened and to allow herself to sit with the pain. She had to accept that she could not change the past and that her anger was still strongly present. Fortunately, radically accepting her

---

Chinese Finger Puzzle

A Chinese finger puzzle, also known as a Chinese finger trap, is a toy used to play a practical joke on someone. You ask a friend to put his or her index fingers into the openings at each end of the little woven straw tube that comprises the puzzle. Once the fingers are inserted, you ask your friend to pull them out. The harder your friend pulls, the tighter the soft material of the tube closes around the now trapped fingers. The only way to free the fingers is to push them toward each other within the tube, which loosens the trap and allows the fingers to slide free.

anger and hurt and expressing these feelings to her husband gave him room to validate her feelings, helping them reestablish needed trust.

Radical acceptance is accepting all of the feelings that come along with a given situation and focusing attention on what can be changed. Radical acceptance does not require forgiveness or generosity of spirit—although these may follow. One thing we often hear from our patients is that they experience less suffering after they've practiced radically accepting their emotions. They explain that while they still feel the pain and distress of their difficult emotions, these pass more quickly because they are not fighting or struggling against them. Imagine a 3-year-old child who has fallen down, skinned her knee, and is crying loudly. Would you sternly tell that 3-year-old child to stop crying? If you did, most 3-year-olds would cry all the more, their pain turned to suffering due to being met with disapproval and an absence of comfort. Accepting that she is sad and scared is the first step to helping calm down this crying child. Radically accepting your emotions allows you to meet your inner 3-year-old where he or she is. Similar to accepting the crying child's tears, acknowledging and accepting your distress makes it more likely your emotions will pass, since you aren't engaged in a battle to deny or resist them. This may free you to make a more effective choice than to binge and allows you to focus on the actual, underlying problem.

Take some time to practice radically accepting your emotions using the following exercise.

EXERCISE 3 Practicing Radically Accepting Your Emotions
in an Imaginary Situation

For the first few times you practice radically accepting your emotions, it can be helpful to remind yourself of situations that you already have experience accepting, such as a natural phenomenon like the weather. Practicing radically accepting your emotions is not that different from accepting you will get wet if you step into the rain without an umbrella. In a fundamental way, you are able to accept that the situation is exactly as it is meant to be, given that it is raining and you have nothing to keep yourself dry. You do not have to like or approve of the fact that you will get wet to be able to radically accept being wet. This exercise builds on this principle to help you gain practice in what it means to radically accept your emotions.

"Begin by imagining that you have planned a very special outdoor occasion to which you have invited your friends and family (e.g., a party, wedding, or a graduation). Now imagine that it is raining on that day. While your emotion about this situation may be stronger than when you're stepping out into the rain on any other day, remember that the principle behind accepting your emotion is the same as the principle behind accepting the weather or other natural phenomenon. Put another way, refusing to accept your emotion is like telling yourself you're not soaked from the rain. You could insist, but the facts are that your head is still getting wet and that is annoying, disappointing, and uncomfortable.

"Now practice radically accepting your emotions (disappointment, irritation, etc.) in the imaginary situation of having it rain on a special outdoor occasion. Practice observing your emotions and adopting a nonjudgmental stance. Each time you find yourself trying to push away or avoid your experience, remind yourself that the emotional sensation is like the sensation of rain on your head during a storm or that of the heat on your face from the sun—sensations that make up your current reality."

In the space below, briefly describe whether you were able to practice radically accepting your emotions in the imaginary situation.

_____

_____

_____

_____

_____

_____

Kat wrote:

I was able to radically accept my disappointment when I imagined I was singing at a friend's wedding and it got rained out. I found the image of accepting my emotions like I would accept rain making me physically wet to be helpful.

Once you have a sense that you understand radically accepting a not-too-intense emotion, you should be ready for the next exercise, which involves an opportunity to practice this skill with an emotion that is more intense.

EXERCISE 4 Practicing Radically Accepting Your Emotions about a Situation You Have Difficulty Accepting

"Begin by thinking of a situation or some fact about your life that you are having difficulty accepting. Practice observing the emotion that comes up as you review the details of the situation and the distress that it causes. Make a decision, when you are ready, to practice radically accepting your emotions. While observing your emotion, deliberately adopt a nonjudgmental stance, allowing yourself to accept whatever your emotion is, even if it is painful and you wish you did not feel it. Notice any urge to make your emotion go away or avoid it—yet allow it to be just what it is. Tell yourself that your emotion is valid and is a part of your experience. Even emotions that are painful or that we judge as unacceptable can have meaning and lead to wisdom. The skill of radically accepting allows you to accept your emotion's presence instead of using food to try to avoid or block experiencing it. Perhaps you can think of times in the past when, looking back, you wish you had accepted your emotion instead of turning to food, which only led to greater suffering. Apply your new understanding about the importance of radically accepting your emotions to your current situation.

"While breathing in and out for 10 breaths, continue to practice radically accepting your emotion at its root. Then end the exercise."

In the space below, describe the situation and your experience with practicing radically accepting your emotions regarding this situation.

_____

_____

_____

_____

_____

_____

_____

_____

_____

_____

_____

_____

_____

_____

_____

_____

_____

Kat wrote:

The situation I am picturing is the day after I had a conversation with my husband asking him not to bring food home that he gets as gifts from his clients. That next evening he came in the door with a package of a dozen French macaroons of all different colors and flavors. I thought: "His behavior is totally unacceptable! He's completely insensitive!" Intense rage started to flow inside of me. This triggered incredible anxiety, because I find it so scary to be angry, so I shoved my feelings down inside me and didn't say anything to him. I started to feel detached and numb. I threw out the food the next day and felt numb, though I knew I must still be angry because he hates when food is wasted. I didn't want to remind him of what I had asked him to do. I just wanted to stay withdrawn.

So I decided for this exercise to practice radically accepting the situation and my anger. I reviewed the details of that evening, thinking back on what I felt in my body when I saw what he had brought home. I brought it back in my mind, observing my heart starting to pound and my muscles tensing and my urge to scream at him. Then I noticed an urge to clamp down on those feelings and a self-judgment that I would turn into a "rage-aholic" like my father if I didn't forgive my husband. So for this exercise, I practiced adopting a nonjudgmental stance and told myself that I can accept this situation and I can accept my anger. And that just because I am angry doesn't mean I will do something out of control. I tried to say to myself, "It's OK to feel the way I am feeling, all feelings pass." As I write this, it's amazing how much calmer I feel. When I let myself be human, accepting that I have emotions that are hard, they really do pass more quickly. I don't have to push these feelings away; I can sit with them, because they are valid. In the past I would have binged on those macaroons for sure and avoided talking to my husband for quite a while. I'd also be certain he had deliberately brought the macaroons home because I'm not important enough for him to do what I'd asked him to and stop bringing food home. Now I'm calm enough to be willing to find out if maybe he just forgot our conversation from the day before. He's been bringing home his clients' gifts for so long, it's really become a habit. I may need to help him remember.

Chapter 9 Summary

This chapter focused on two skills to improve how you deal with intense emotions: mindfulness of your current emotion and radically accepting your emotions. Increasing your ability to skillfully cope with intense emotion makes you less likely to turn to binge eating.

Mindfulness of your current emotion uses observing as well as adopting a nonjudgmental stance and focusing on one thing in this moment to pay attention to emotions in their entirety. Instead of judging yourself for having the painful emotion, which makes the emotion stronger, this skill allows the emotion to decrease naturally and change over time. This skill is similar to urge surfing except instead of letting the urge to binge eat pass, one lets the intense emotion pass.

Sometimes it can be particularly difficult to become fully aware of an emotion. You may be tempted to push the emotion away and bury it with food. The second skill discussed in this chapter, radically accepting your emotions, involves accepting your emotions in a deep and fundamental way. It does not require approving of them. But in accepting your emotions instead of fighting their existence, you can turn your attention toward determining what you may be able to change about the situation that is causing the emotion and at the same time accepting what you cannot change.

We asked you to complete several exercises to practice both of these skills. As you become more familiar with these skills you will become better able to deal with strong emotions and be more able to live according to your wise mind.

Homework

Remember to check the box after you have completed each homework assignment.

HOMEWORK EXERCISE 9-A

Practicing Being Mindful of Your Current Emotion
This Coming Week

Practice being mindful of your current emotion every day this week. Use the mindfulness skills of observing, adopting a nonjudgmental stance, and focusing on one thing in this moment. Remind yourself, especially when experiencing particularly powerful emotions, of past emotions you felt "stuck" in at the time but that no longer feel so powerful. Remind yourself that your current state of mind and your current emotion are just what you are experiencing in this present moment. Describe your practice of the skill below (using additional pages as necessary).

_____

_____

_____

_____

_____

_____

_____

❑ I have practiced mindfulness of my current emotions every day this week, and I have written about the experience above.

HOMEWORK EXERCISE 9-B
Radical Acceptance, Letting Go of Emotional Suffering

At least three times this week, practice letting go of emotional suffering by radically accepting your emotions, particularly when you are experiencing urges to binge eat. Accept the emotion and the situation, and turn toward it instead of away from it. Describe your practice of this skill to replace problem eating behaviors (using additional pages as necessary).

_____

_____

_____

_____

_____

_____

_____

_____

_____

_____

_____

❑ I have practiced the skill, radically accepting your emotions, at least three times this week and written about this experience in the space provided.

❑ I have filled out my Diary Card daily.

❑ I have filled out at least one Behavioral Chain Analysis Form this week.

❑ I have used the skills I find most helpful so that I can use my wise mind and stop binge eating before it happens.

10

Reducing Vulnerability to Emotion Mind and Building Mastery

The rationale for teaching the skills in this chapter is that you are more likely to binge eat when you are in emotion mind. The skills of diaphragmatic breathing, dialectical thinking, and observing can help you shift from your emotion mind to your wise mind. Now we offer skills that can reduce your vulnerability to being in emotion mind in the first place.

Decreasing Vulnerability to Emotion Mind

EXERCISE 1 Identifying Connections between Specific Vulnerability Factors and Binge Eating

Have you noticed that when you're tired, ill, extremely hungry, or otherwise stretched or stressed you're more emotionally reactive, more likely to have urges to turn to food to self-soothe, and more likely to binge eat? Identifying the specific factors related to your lifestyle and environment that increase your vulnerability to your emotion mind is the first step to changing these factors. Review your most recent behavioral chain analyses and then, in the space below, **list typical vulnerabilities from Section 3 of your Behavioral Chain Analysis Forms.** Don't worry if you had difficulty identifying very many. Through the rest of this chapter, we'll be helping you focus on common environmental/lifestyle vulnerabilities and what you can do to address them.

_____

_____

_____

_____

_____

_____

_____

_____

_____

_____

Kat wrote:

I reviewed my past behavioral chain analyses. What I've noticed are two main vulnerabilities. One is fatigue. I'm definitely more vulnerable to my emotion mind and more likely to have difficulty controlling my binge eating when I'm tired. Most of my binge eating tends to occur late at night. Getting more sleep would help me because I'd be less tired, but also going to sleep earlier would reduce the amount of time I'd be awake in the late evening.

The second factor is an intense emotional state, feeling chronically lonely and hopeless. I am much more vulnerable to my emotion mind when I'm overwhelmed by those feelings. It seems to be something I wake up with and can't shake off. It makes me want to avoid doing anything I don't absolutely have to do and just stay home with my cat and dogs.

The PLEASE Acronym to Reduce Vulnerability to Emotion Mind

The acronym PLEASE

- Treat PhysicaL illness.

- Balance your Eating.

- Avoid mood-altering substances.

- Balance your Sleep.

- Get Exercise.

can help you remember five ways to reduce common environmental/lifestyle factors that make you vulnerable to your emotion mind. As we review each area, we will ask you to think about how it may apply to you. Clearly, some factors will be more relevant than others. Of these, we will help you think about which ones you can change and what steps you're willing to take to do so.

TREAT PHYSICAL ILLNESS

John was raised to go to school regardless of how he was feeling physically. He had perfect attendance as a child—but that simply meant that his parents did not keep him home unless he was so ill he needed to go to the hospital. He was taught the importance of a "stiff upper lip." As with his emotions, his physical health was often ignored.

As an adult, John continued to not pay attention to his body and rarely if ever called in sick. He ignored body aches, colds, feeling run down—he just kept his "stiff upper lip" and "soldiered on." When John's body sent him messages that he was sick, he ignored the information—just as he had ignored his emotions before he started this program. But attempting to ignore signals of being run down, achy, and physically unwell did not make the symptoms better. Instead, by pushing himself to function when he was sick, he felt more stressed, more irritable, and more emotionally reactive. He was much more vulnerable to his emotion mind. When he made mistakes, which was more common in this state, he judged himself even more harshly than usual. This made him more prone to guilt and shame—increasing the likelihood he would binge eat.

When he recognized the role of physical illness in his vulnerability to binge eating on his Behavioral Chain Analysis Forms, John started—for the first time—to take sick days when he was ill. He began to listen to his body and give it what it needed when it needed it. As a result he didn't feel spread so thin, and now he could focus on getting well and not continue to push himself beyond what he was capable of. This decreased his sense of shame and guilt about being less productive, making him less vulnerable to urges to binge eat.

Do you try to ignore your body's messages when you're feeling sick so as to be able to function "the same as always?"

Yes No

Do you notice patterns of turning to food when you are feeling physically unwell?

Yes No

EXERCISE 2   How Does Ignoring Physical Illness Affect Your
                Emotional Vulnerability and Binge Eating?

a. Many people who binge eat have a tendency to distract themselves from
noticing their body's signals. When they actually do take the time to pay
attention to themselves, they often admit they are more likely to feel anxious or irritable when they are sick. These feelings can make it harder to
manage stressful situations appropriately and can lower their resistance to
binge eating. Is this true for you as well? Discuss in the space provided how
tendencies you may have to ignore physical illness are related to greater
emotional vulnerability and an increased likelihood of binge eating. Use an
extra page if needed.

_____

_____

_____

_____

Kat wrote:

I hate being sick and am a terrible patient. So this is true of me. I think
I've gotten better as I've gotten older, though. I've had to because I just
can't ignore my body when it is sick like I used to. I definitely am more
vulnerable to my emotion mind when I'm sick. I feel more needy, and if
Tom doesn't seem sympathetic I easily feel angry at him and feel sorry
for myself. I often don't know how or don't even want to ask him for
the extra attention and care I want. Though it's not so true now, in the
past I definitely found it a lot easier to turn to food to soothe myself.

b. If you do tend to ignore physical illness, what changes in your behavior
would you be willing to make when you're physically ill to reduce this source
of vulnerability?

_____

_____

_____

_____

Kat wrote:

My commitment to stop binge eating feels very strong to me now.
Recognizing how ignoring physical illness makes me more vulnerable,

I am certainly willing to not push myself when I'm physically ill. But I also need to stop delaying. Sometimes I wait too long—only making a doctor's appointment, for instance, when the pain in my shoulder is so bad that I can't move it instead of going a week earlier when it was just starting to really hurt. I deserve to be careful with my body—it's the only one I have.

BALANCE YOUR **E**ATING

Although she didn't really want to admit it, Leticia had to agree that diets didn't really seem to work for her. She had been on so many over the years and yet was never "done." She was always starting another one, it seemed. The fact that thousands of diets are constantly being created by the diet industry was pretty good evidence to her that none of them really worked in the long run. Intellectually, she understood this and knew she was not alone. She also understood that many of her habits ended up setting her up to binge eat—habits like trying to lose weight quickly, trying to eat very little during the day so that she could "save" calories for a dinner out (such as a meal at her mother's home), and often attempting to cut out certain foods (e.g., all sweets). Prolonged food restriction would make her so hungry that her physical urges to eat became more intense, making her feel uncomfortable and irritable. She was more vulnerable to being in emotion mind by the time she eventually ate. Then, if she ate more than she had planned, she was more likely to feel demoralized and to binge. Although she understood this pattern wasn't working, accepting this was incredibly difficult for her. And accepting that she would most likely stay at her current weight was also very hard. Of all her eating challenges, accepting her weight and stopping her constant attempts to diet/restrict her eating were the hardest. Eventually, and with great effort, over time she was able to use radical acceptance to acknowledge that she needed to stop restricting her eating so severely. Ultimately, she was able to use this skill to put into action something she already knew deep down inside—that she needed to balance her eating. She created a meal plan for herself instead of restricting during the day and risking being in emotion mind at night and therefore being so vulnerable to binge eating. She was thankful, but not surprised, when she noticed a drop in her binge urges once she was eating regularly and no longer hungry during the day.

It is common for those who binge eat to attempt to diet. Such attempts can include trying to limit the overall amount of food you eat, attempting to avoid eating particular foods (e.g., sweets, carbohydrates, fats), and/or attempting to fast for long periods of time. Research shows that just attempting to follow a restrictive diet, whether or not you actually "succeed," increases the likelihood that you will binge eat. Putting effort into losing weight through restrictive dieting actually *contributes* to binge eating and thus to weight gain. And years of data show that diets very rarely lead to maintained weight loss. Most people regain the weight they lost, and many gain even more.

We strongly recommend that patients who come to us work on stopping binge eating do not simultaneously attempt to lose weight. This is the same recommendation we gave in the Introduction. There are several important reasons for this advice. One is that when people who binge are put on a diet, they often find that the rigid structure and rules help them stop binge eating—*but only temporarily.* You may have noticed this too. The problem with diets is that most people who diet will regain the weight they lost. For people who binge eat, the chances that this will happen are even greater. Binge eaters are at much higher risk of being "yo-yo" dieters.

Dieting during this program can rob you of the opportunity to apply the skills taught because they wouldn't be needed while your binge eating had stopped temporarily. Then, once you'd finished the program, your risk of regaining the weight would be very high because you wouldn't really have learned how to stop binge eating. Regaining the weight would be very demoralizing, and in response you might decide to discard whatever skills you had learned, believing that this program was one more thing that didn't work for your binge eating. This is why we want you to focus primarily and directly on binge eating.

Another reason we do not recommend trying to lose weight while working through this program is that dieting is very stressful and requires a great deal of focus. For example, losing weight involves shopping for low-calorie foods, taking time to prepare them, cook them, exercise, and so forth. It's very difficult to concentrate both on dieting and on doing all the reading and exercises involved in this program.

As already mentioned, another difficulty with dieting is the possibility that the rigid rules boomerang and, instead of finding that the structure decreases your binge eating, you become more vulnerable to your emotion mind (due to greater physical hunger, greater emotional stress, getting stuck and giving up once you break a "rule") and thus even more likely to binge eat and gain weight.

We want to reiterate that we understand that weight loss may be your goal. We want to make sure you are aware that the available research suggests you'll be more likely to lose weight and keep the weight off (which is the ultimate challenge) if you first eliminate binge eating. In fact, some weight loss often accompanies cessation of bingeing. This is also why our program focuses on stopping binge eating and not weight loss, at least until the elimination of binge eating has been achieved.

If you use your new skills to stop binge eating and remain binge free by the end of this program, you and your physician will be in a much better position to have an effective discussion about potential weight loss. In consultation with your wise mind, you might consider issues such as whether or not remaining binge abstinent will ultimately lead to sufficient weight loss (data indicate losses of about 5–10% of one's body weight) to meet your "wellness" goals. Also, it would be important to consider whether reintroducing a focus on weight loss, especially if done too quickly, might threaten your hard-won binge abstinence. The bottom line is that choosing to pursue weight loss is a complex topic. The skills that help you stop binge eating, such as dialectical thinking and adopting a nonjudgmental stance, will help you navigate your future options as wisely as possible.

A different pattern that characterizes some binge eaters is *excessive eating between binge episodes*. This pattern also increases vulnerability to emotion mind and thus binge eating because taking in too many calories above what your body requires leads to short-term consequences like sluggishness, nausea, and head-aches, as well as long-term consequences from obesity, including arthritis, cardio-vascular disease, sleep apnea, and diabetes.

Balanced eating involves neither restricting nor overeating. The United States Department of Agriculture (USDA) offers tips on balanced eating based on the five food groups (grains, dairy, fruit, vegetables, protein). See Choose My Plate at *www.choosemyplate.gov*.

To reiterate, stopping binge eating is the best way to stop gaining weight over time and to increase your chances of experiencing sustained weight loss.

Have there been periods when you tried to restrict what you eat and/or are you currently attempting to restrict what you eat?

> Yes   No

Have there been periods when you ate excessively between your binge episodes and/or are you currently doing so?

> Yes   No

EXERCISE 3   How Does Imbalanced Eating Affect Your Emotional Vulnerability and Binge Eating?

a. What relationship are you aware of—either directly or over time—between times that your eating is out of balance, through restrictive dieting and/or eating excessively between binge episodes, and your experience of greater emotional vulnerability and likelihood of binge eating? Explain in the space provided, using an extra page if needed.

_____

_____

_____

_____

_____

_____

_____

_____

_____

_____

_____

_____

_____

_____

_____

_____

_____

_____

Kat wrote:

I have a tendency to try to restrict my eating—especially when I am feeling fat. I try to lose weight quickly by trying to starve myself for a day or two despite already noticing how that leads me to binge. What I never quite understood was that starving myself didn't just make me feel super hungry—though it did. It also made me emotionally vulnerable because I was irritable and crabby and cranky. In other words, in emotion mind. I was hypersensitive to Tom—easily felt hurt. I'd give him the silent treatment when he wouldn't say the right thing, and my emotion mind would tell me this was justified. Also, after a couple of days of trying to practically starve, I always broke down and ate more than the little bit I'd allowed myself. It might just be a small extra serving of nuts—really nothing much at all, but it was often on the same day I felt like I hadn't moved at all because I'd been so tired from not eating enough. So my emotion mind would tell me that I was lazy and

I'd feel guilty and ashamed because I had messed up and the day was "ruined." Emotion mind was so rigid—I couldn't even think straight. It was worse because I was genuinely starved. I'd have a full-out binge, avoid Tom, and end up going to sleep really late, feeling sick and hung over and miserable. I didn't want to wake up the next day.

b. If you have noticed that a lack of balance in your eating is related to greater emotional vulnerability and an increased likelihood of binge eating, **describe below how you plan to begin to balance your eating patterns, starting now.**

_____

_____

_____

_____

_____

_____

_____

_____

_____

_____

_____

_____

_____

_____

_____

Kat wrote:

I know that I have to give up my focus on weight loss. Reading this chapter has helped. I know diets don't work. I just really need to practice radical acceptance. Trying to lose weight quickly through crash dieting has never been helpful for me, and to gain control of my weight I need to focus on stopping binge eating and letting myself follow normal guidelines for eating rather than an overly strict food plan that I know I am never truly going to be able to stick to. I am willing to make a change by eating breakfast. That is a meal I skip—partly because, at least in the past, I overate at night and was not that hungry in the morning. But these days I have kept it up even if I overeat at night. Though I am not really overweight, I hate the feeling of my eating being out of control. And as I get older, I feel I just gain weight so much more easily that I want to skip calories wherever I can. But it really sets me up to be in emotion mind and over the long run, even if not immediately, this will set me up to binge. And I do not want this vulnerability. My quality of life is too important to me, and my commitment to stop binge eating and stay stopped is so vital to all that I value.

AVOID/REDUCE MOOD-ALTERING SUBSTANCES

Mood-altering substances, including illegal as well as legal drugs, certain prescription medications, caffeine, nicotine, and alcohol, can influence your emotional state and cloud your ability to think clearly about your choices. This can make you more vulnerable to your emotion mind and increase the likelihood that you will binge eat. Answer the following questions and reflect on how various mood-altering substances may be affecting you.

Do you react to caffeine by becoming more agitated and less calm?

Yes   No

Does alcohol make you more emotionally vulnerable?

Yes   No

Are you more likely to binge eat after drinking alcohol?

Yes   No

If you use other mood-altering substances, like marijuana, are you more likely to binge or emotionally eat during or after using them?

Yes   No

EXERCISE 4 How Do Mood-Altering Substances Affect Your Relationship with Emotional Vulnerability and Binge Eating?

a. Write about **your use of mood-altering substances.** Is there a relationship that links your use of them with your **vulnerability to your emotion mind and binge eating?** If so, how important is it to you to address this?

_____
_____
_____
_____
_____
_____
_____
_____

Kat wrote:

My problem is caffeine. I drink about three cups throughout the morning so I am less hungry. It makes it easier to skip breakfast and sometimes other meals when I am trying to starve for a couple of days. So
this relates to what I wrote about balanced eating, too. But it's its own
problem because it doesn't just stop me from being hungry. It makes
me jittery and antsy and more stressed. I never really thought about
it as making me more vulnerable to emotion mind, but that helps me
be more willing to lower my consumption, along with realizing I have
to eat breakfast anyway. I think the combination of being hungry and
being amped up on caffeine definitely makes me more emotionally vulnerable and eventually leads me to be more likely to binge.

b. **What changes in your use of mood-altering substances would you be
willing to make to reduce this source of vulnerability?**

_____
_____
_____
_____
_____
_____
_____

Kat wrote:

I drink A LOT of coffee in the morning so that I don't eat till lunch. So I am willing to replace ¼ of my caffeinated coffee with decaf starting tomorrow morning, and to stay that way for 1 week. Then the next week I am willing to go to half caffeine, half decaf. I've never really tried to do this before, but I've heard of other people gradually lowering the amount of caffeine this way. If I have withdrawal, I'll slow it down, but otherwise I should be at full decaf in 1 month from now. I think my reasons for using caffeine are about my weight and that if I want coffee I can have decaf, with coffee on special occasions when I am having a meal anyway (not to try to skip a meal, like now).

BALANCE YOUR **S**LEEP

Sleep is essential for emotional stability. When our bodies are tired, our emotional vulnerability is heightened. Instead of dealing directly with fatigue, for example, by going to sleep earlier or taking a nap, individuals often use food to increase energy. The use of extra food, coupled with emotional vulnerability, can even further increase the likelihood of a binge.

Just as not getting enough sleep can increase vulnerability to emotion mind, so can sleeping too much (e.g., averaging more than 9 hours per night). Oversleeping can be caused by medical conditions (e.g., sleep apnea, depression, and diabetes) as well as by certain substances (e.g., alcohol, prescription drugs). The consequences of oversleeping, both physical (e.g., back pain, headaches, feeling overtired) and emotional (e.g., waking up anxious, being self-critical, feeling more depressed), can increase vulnerability to emotion mind.

Does having unbalanced sleep make you more vulnerable to your emotion mind and hence to binge eating?

Yes   No

Do you attempt to overcome tiredness by eating food to increase your energy rather than responding more directly to being tired?

Yes   No

EXERCISE 5 How Does Imbalanced Sleep Affect Your Emotional Vulnerability and Binge Eating?

a. In the space below, describe any relationships you are aware of that link **your sleep patterns (getting too little or too much sleep) with being more emotionally vulnerable and at greater risk for binge eating.**

_____

_____

_____

_____

_____

_____

_____

_____

_____

_____

Kat wrote:

I sleep too little, but also, at times, I oversleep. I never really thought about oversleeping as making me more vulnerable to my emotion mind, but I can see that it is true. I feel awful when I oversleep. Usually it's when I drink alcohol or stay up too late binge eating (I can see how these vulnerability factors often become related to each other). When I do that, I wake up feeling guilty and upset at myself. It really starts my day off so that I'm very vulnerable. I feel ashamed, like I've wasted half the day already. It takes very little for me to find some excuse from emotion mind to set me off toward binge eating.

   Not getting enough sleep the night before makes me particularly vulnerable in the evening—when I am most likely to binge. Going to sleep earlier would be very helpful.

b. How important is it to you to address **balancing your sleep** to lower your risk of emotional vulnerability and binge eating? **What changes in your sleep patterns would you be willing to make** to reduce this source of vulnerability to binge eating?

_____

_____

_____

_____

_____

_____

_____

_____

_____

Kat wrote:

I never really understood before how destructive oversleeping was in making me more vulnerable to my emotion mind like I do now. I really feel willing to work on going to sleep earlier, although it feels like I am starting to try to make too many changes all at the same time. But I do know it is important. So maybe going to sleep just 15 minutes earlier. Even that would make a difference. The oversleeping is less frequent. The change I need to make there is to cut down on drinking. That is something I didn't think of in that section. That really is not that hard for me.

GET EXERCISE

Lack of exercise can also be a source of emotional vulnerability, leading to an overall decreased sense of physical stamina and lack of emotional well-being. Physical inactivity can increase your vulnerability to depression and to emotion mind and can increase your chances of binge eating. Becoming more physically active, on the other hand, can be a very effective way to improve your mood, reduce your stress, and increase your overall level of functioning. Getting exercise, especially for people with a tendency toward binge eating when they're depressed, can be a particularly helpful tool.

Research overwhelmingly supports increasing your activity level as one of the most effective ways to improve your mood, especially when you are feeling down or discouraged. An important feature of exercise is that it acts independently of your mood. In other words, you don't need to be in a good mood to exercise. Exercise will act to change your mood! In turn, this will reduce your vulnerability to your emotion mind and the likelihood that you will binge.

It is important to note that getting moderate exercise does not require running a marathon or pushing yourself to the point of injury! It means, in a balanced way, doing something to get your limbs moving, such as walking, swimming, or bicycling. The focus is on balanced, moderate exercise.

While increased activity is important, it is also essential to distinguish this from overexercise. Overexercise, or exercising to excess, includes compulsively exercising without adequate rest or nourishment, and/or exercising despite being injured. Overexercise causes physical and emotional imbalance and stress, which increase your vulnerability to emotion mind and thus to binge eating. As briefly discussed in the Introduction and in Chapter 3, however, sometimes overexercise itself is what individuals turn to, instead of binge eating, as a way of avoiding or escaping emotional discomfort. Overexercise can increase the likelihood of binge eating because when you turn to overexercise to avoid emotional discomfort, you lose an opportunity to use a healthy skill to manage your emotions—thus strengthening the link you wish to break between feeling distress and turning to an unhealthy behavior out of line with your core values.

Reflect on your own experiences with physical activity. Have you noticed that it can affect your mood?

Yes   No

Are you more likely to be emotionally vulnerable when you are not getting enough exercise or, alternatively, when you are overexercising?

Yes   No

Do you have a regular exercise program?

Yes   No

EXERCISE 6   How Does Physical Activity Affect Your Emotional Vulnerability and Binge Eating?

a. **Write about your use of exercise or physical activity.** Is there a relationship between your use of physical activity, your emotional vulnerability, and your likelihood of binge eating?

_____

_____

_____

_____

_____

_____

_____

_____

_____

Kat wrote:

Overexercise is definitely not my problem. Right now, though, I am reasonably active because I use public transportation and have to walk quite a bit between stops. This gives me enough activity to make me feel I move around during the day. Also, although I also didn't see it mentioned in the list of activities, I garden. That feels like a good amount of activity for someone my age. It's not too strenuous, but with planting, pruning, deadheading the spent blooms, watering, etc., it's a lot. I definitely notice that I feel much better and in a better mood on days that I'm more physically active and I am less vulnerable to my emotion mind. I am more centered and less likely to be hypersensitive to Tom, more likely to appreciate beauty and the good things in my life that I really enjoy, like singing.

b. If there is a connection, **what changes in your exercise behaviors would you be willing to make to reduce this source of vulnerability?**

_____

_____

_____

_____

_____

_____

_____

_____

_____

_____

_____

Kat wrote:

I never really thought about the role that regular physical activity plays. Thinking about it now, I would certainly be willing to make sure I don't go long periods without it. I only garden part of the year, so in the winter I'd be willing to do more walking. It would definitely be worth it. I like the idea of it being mood independent. I need to remember that I don't have to feel like walking to do it. I can be in a bad mood and in fact it will help me—even though when I am in a bad mood the last thing I want to do is move. I want to mope and eat. But it helps me to think of it as mood independent and as a way to reduce my vulnerability to emotion mind. I am someone who is more likely to binge when I'm depressed, so physical activity is important for me to do regularly. It's worth anything to reduce my emotional vulnerability. A small cost compared to the huge cost and dead-end life that I have if I can't keep my commitment to myself to stop binge eating and turn to this program first.

Building Mastery

Building mastery involves doing activities that increase your sense of competence and confidence. Feeling more satisfied and fulfilled makes you less vulnerable to painful or negative emotions such as depression and increases the likelihood of experiencing pleasant emotions.

To build mastery, you need to identify activities that require some effort, are somewhat challenging, and help you build self-esteem and satisfaction. Actually engaging in these confidence-enhancing behaviors each day (not just thinking about them) gives new and different feedback to your brain, helping to change your emotional experience. Like exercise, any form of building mastery is a mood-independent behavior. Activities that promote building mastery might include doing something creative, like playing music, writing, or engaging in crafts, as well as learning a new language, taking a course, or reading a challenging book. Especially for people who binge eat, exercising is an excellent activity for building mastery.

Do you think enhancing a sense of mastery would help decrease your vulnerability to your emotion mind, making you less likely to binge eat?

Yes   No

EXERCISE 7   How Does Building Mastery Affect Your Emotional
Vulnerability and Binge Eating?

a. **Write about experiences of mastery in your life.** Is there a relationship
between not having enough mastery experiences, your vulnerability to
emotion mind, and binge eating? If there is a relationship, how important is
it to you to address this factor?

_____

_____

_____

_____

_____

_____

_____

Kat wrote:

I think that while I do have experiences of mastery that make me
feel good about myself, I don't really take them in. I perform through
my singing and I am constantly involved in creative, meaningful work.
But I am always critiquing myself, always trying to be better. Maybe I
need to find something that I DO feel more confident about. I need to
think about this. One of the things I truly enjoy is making jewelry, and
I haven't done that for years. To me it is something I've done just for
fun—never anything I'd try to sell. But I do love it. I would have to say
that there is a relationship between not having enough mastery experiences and being more vulnerable to emotion mind and binge eating
because I've been involved in the arts for a long time and have binged
through most of that time. So it clearly wasn't giving me enough of that
sense of competence.

b. **List some activities that would build mastery** for you.

_____

_____

_____

_____

_____

Kat wrote:

I am thinking that jewelry making would build mastery. I also enjoy playing music. I've always wanted to play the piano, and I'm thinking that if I started to take lessons I would feel a sense of mastery simply from that. It would be a huge accomplishment for so many reasons. A way of growing, a challenge, a risk. I'd feel so proud of myself for start- ing something new. I've also always wanted to take a conversational Spanish class. Any of these would help me build mastery.

c. If you feel that you do not have enough opportunities in your life to build mastery and accomplishment, **make a plan to engage in some of the activities** you listed to help build your confidence. Write your plan in the space provided, using extra paper if needed.

_____

_____

_____

_____

_____

_____

Kat wrote:

I think the way to start would be for me to start making jewelry again. I have a lot of the materials already. I just have to go back to it. I also think it's time I learned to play the piano. We actually have an upright. Maybe the first step is to get it tuned. Then I can ask around about teachers in the area that are good.

d. As we mentioned above, each of the six areas we have discussed (e.g., treat physical illness, balance your eating, avoid mood-altering substances, balance your sleep, get exercise, and build mastery) involve ways to reduce your vulnerability to your emotion mind and thus also reduce your suscep- tibility to binge eating. It's likely that other factors are missing from our discussion that also make you vulnerable to emotion mind. If so, name the factors and write down a plan to reduce your vulnerability to them in the space below.

_____

_____

_____

_____

_____

_____

_____

_____

_____

_____

_____

_____

_____

_____

_____

Kat wrote:

One of my vulnerabilities includes the influence of bad habits. This wasn't mentioned in the chapter. There is something about habits and routines that makes me want to do the same thing again—makes me feel almost like I have to do the same thing again, just because I did it the day before. It can get me into cycles where I can binge for weeks at a time, and it starts to feel like there really is no prompting event that day because nothing really happened except for the fact that I had binged the day before. So one of the things I need to do is to change routines that are harmful to me. If I have a day that I binge and oversleep and feel terrible, I need to find a way to get out and exercise or do something that increases my sense of mastery. I need to do something that changes the pattern. If I don't, and just do the "same old same old," I will get the "same old same old" back.

Chapter 10 Summary

This chapter discussed ways to reduce your vulnerability to your emotion mind, which ultimately will help decrease behaviors such as binge eating. A total of six different environmental/lifestyle factors were discussed. To remember five of them, we used the acronym PLEASE, which stands for:

- Treat **P**hysica**L** illness
- Balance your **E**ating
- **A**void mood-altering substances
- Balance your **S**leep
- Get **E**xercise

Treating physical illness, eating a well-balanced diet, and being well rested were listed as factors that can help you feel less run down and more able to shift from your emotion mind to your wise mind, and thus help you cope with negative moods that do occur.

This chapter also discussed how mood-altering substances, by increasing your emotional vulnerability, make it harder to access your wise mind and increase the likelihood of a binge. Two final factors were discussed: getting exercise and building mastery. Both of these mood-independent behaviors also help decrease your emotional vulnerability and susceptibility to binge eating.

This chapter included exercises asking you to think about the degree to which these six factors affected you and to make plans to decrease your vulnerability to them. Working to decrease your vulnerability factors will not only decrease binge eating but also increase your overall life satisfaction (which we think is always a good thing!).

Homework

Remember to check the box after you have completed each homework assignment.

HOMEWORK EXERCISE 10-A

Filling out the Worksheet "Steps for Reducing Vulnerability to Emotion Mind" over the Following Week

Use the worksheet "Steps for Reducing Vulnerability to Emotion Mind" on the facing page to make specific plans for each of the six environmental/lifestyle factors listed. (See the end of the Contents for information on printing out additional copies.) For example, if too little sleep is a problem, you might make it a goal to get at least 8 hours of sleep for 5 of the next 7 days. Circle the days you actually put your plans into action. Although the worksheet focuses on how

Steps for Reducing Vulnerability to Emotion Mind

For each factor, write down your specific plan to reduce your vulnerability to your emotion mind over the week. Circle the day(s) you actually put your plans into action and describe what took place.

Reducing Vulnerability to Emotion Mind

Treat physical illness?

Plan: _____

_____

M T W Th F S Sun

Outcome: _____

_____

Balance your eating?

Plan: _____

_____

M T W Th F S Sun

Outcome: _____

_____

Avoid mood-altering substances?

Plan: _____

_____

M T W Th F S Sun

Outcome: _____

_____

Balance your sleep?

Plan: _____

_____

M T W Th F S Sun

Outcome: _____

_____

Get exercise?

Plan: _____

_____

M T W Th F S Sun

Outcome: _____

_____

Practice building mastery?

Plan: _____

_____

M T W Th F S Sun

Outcome: _____

_____

you put these plans into action over the next week, the goal is to follow these plans throughout the rest of treatment and beyond. Not only will addressing these factors lower your vulnerability to emotion mind and binge eating, but it also will improve your overall mood!

❑ I have used the "Steps for Reducing Vulnerability to Emotion Mind" worksheet to make plans to address each of the vulnerability factors.

❑ I have begun to address my major vulnerability factors this week.

❑ I have filled out my Diary Card daily.

❑ I have filled out at least one Behavioral Chain Analysis Form this week.

❑ I have used the skills I find most helpful so that I can use my wise mind and stop binge eating or other problem behaviors before they happen.

11

Building Positive Experiences

STEPS FOR INCREASING POSITIVE EMOTIONS

You will probably not be surprised to hear that research shows that individuals who binge eat are more likely to experience negative moods such as persistent sadness and depression. Maybe this is something you have experienced firsthand. An important way to improve your overall mood and quality of life is to learn the skills we teach in this program as an alternative to seeking comfort in excess food when you're feeling sad or depressed.

But why are binge eaters more likely to have negative moods in the first place? This vulnerability can often be traced to (1) an imbalance of negative and positive activities and (2) an inability to fully experience and focus attention on positive experiences when they occur. Do you think these factors might apply to you?

Before we discuss these in greater detail and tell you what you can to do to change them, answer the following questions:

QUIZ What Role Do Positive Experiences Play in Your Life?

1. Do the number of negative or neutral activities in your life generally outweigh the number of positive ones?

    Yes   No

2. When you engage in planned pleasant activities, do you find you have difficulty fully enjoying them?

    Yes   No

3. Do you notice that you distract yourself from or interrupt your positive emotional experiences with guilt, worry, and/or self-criticism?

    Yes   No

Responding with yes to one or more of these questions may help explain why you tend to have low moods. You might not think much about how often positive experiences are a part of your life, but when you do, it's pretty obvious that having few engaging, rewarding activities or being unable to really enjoy them is not going to leave you feeling very good. So it makes sense to try to add positive experiences and your enjoyment of them to your life.

Building Positive Experiences

If you think you might be missing out on positive experiences, first recognize that a key notion is balance. This means not working all day, every day, but it also means not being on vacation every day. Another important notion is that to reap the rewards of positive experiences in your life you have to accumulate a number of pleasant experiences. We hope you'll feel the effort to make this investment is worthwhile, because we've seen an imbalance in this area make many of our patients more vulnerable to their emotion mind and thus more likely to turn to food when they experience emotional pain or discomfort.

We recommend four methods for shifting the balance of your life toward the positive:

1. Increase your daily pleasant activities.
2. Accumulate positive emotions long term.
3. Attend to your relationships.
4. Avoid avoiding (especially by turning to binge eating as a way to escape distressing emotions).

Increase Your Daily Pleasant Activities

The Pleasant Events Schedule in the box on the facing page is a sampling of activities that can increase your experience of positive events and positive feelings. There are blanks included in the list for you to fill in using your own ideas for positive events or activities. Right now, these don't have to be events you actually engage in, but ones you imagine you might enjoy.

As you can see, many of these activities are fairly simple to do, as are the pleasant activities that Leticia added to create her own list:

Doing crafts (paint-by-numbers)
Browsing in a bookstore

Pleasant Events Schedule

1. Soaking in a bathtub

2. Going on vacation

3. Relaxing

4. Going to a movie at the beginning of the week

5. Laughing

6. Lying in the sun

7. Listening to music

8. Going to a party

9. Arranging flowers

10. Reading a book or magazine

11. Gardening

12. Going hiking

13. Enjoying a cup of tea

14. _____

15. _____

16. _____

17. _____

18. _____

19. _____

20. _____

Reading the newspaper in a coffee shop

Listening to music

Playing the piano

Painting fingernails

Calling an old friend

Increasing the number of positive activities in your life won't likely be easy. We readily acknowledge that, especially in this day and age, there are multiple demands on your time. Prioritizing positive events requires a true dedication to taking care of yourself as part of your commitment to stop binge eating. However, especially if binge eating was one of your few comforts, it is imperative that you develop other ways to soothe yourself. Otherwise you keep yourself vulnerable to binge eating.

What if prioritizing pleasant events simply seems too self-indulgent when there are so many obligations or activities that you simply "have" to do? It may help to think about the safety announcement at the beginning of a flight that instructs you to put on your own oxygen mask before attempting to help others. If you pass out from lack of oxygen, you won't be able to get anything done, let alone help anyone else. Also, remember that, just as brushing your teeth every day can become a habit, so can engaging in pleasant activities. And while you can't take a vacation every day, you *can* make time every day to do something you find pleasant—whether that means making yourself a cup of fragrant tea or giving yourself a moment to relax.

Engaging in positive activities does not guarantee that you will enjoy them, but it certainly increases the odds.

Accumulate Positive Emotions Long Term

In addition to planning to include more positive activities in your daily life, it is valuable to think of longer-term goals that you could set for yourself that would contribute to leading a more satisfying and fulfilling life—a life in line with your values that would bring you more happiness than you have currently. To remind yourself of these values, you may wish to review Exercise 4 ("Identifying Your Values") in Chapter 2.

EXERCISE 1 Building Long-Term Positive Goals

a. Based on your identified values, **describe one or more longer-term goals** that will help you achieve greater life satisfaction. For example, we have had patients develop and follow through on goals to exhibit their art, explore a new career, and follow up on a long-standing interest in taking music lessons.

_____

_____

_____

_____

_____

_____

Kat wrote:

One of my greatest values is to be an authentic person. When my friend was diagnosed with dementia, I withdrew and had great difficulty staying present in the friendship because of deep feelings of loss and because her illness felt so unfair—both to her and to me. It would really bring me pleasure to find a way to remain in her life as a way of honoring how much I have loved her over the years and how much she has meant to me.

b. Write down some **small steps** you'll need to take to begin to reach these goals. For example, if you were interested in starting the piano lessons you've always wanted but never made time for, small steps to get you started might include (1) asking friends and family for recommendations for a teacher; (2) searching the Internet for information on piano teachers and piano lessons; (3) making a list of teachers you could call; (4) narrowing down the list and beginning to call them; (5) arranging a trial lesson with a teacher; (6) if satisfied with this teacher, stopping the search, but if not, returning to the list and continuing to call teachers.

_____

_____

_____

_____

_____

_____

_____

_____

_____

_____

Kat wrote:

Some small steps I can take to reach my goal are:

1. *I can plan to visit my friend at least every 2 weeks.*

2. *I will sing for her regardless of her mental state. I think this will bring her pleasure as she has always loved music.*

3. *To help me stay present and to funnel energy that otherwise might*

go into binge eating, I want to find some way to be creative. This is such a deep value of mine—being able to experience all of what fate brings us and facing that with creativity and authenticity. I am not exactly sure what form this will take. I'm thinking maybe I could write a song about this experience.

Attend to Your Relationships

Most people value having good relationships and see these as an essential component of a meaningful life. Many of our patients report that their binge eating has interfered with their ability to work on their current relationships, set boundaries in relationships that feel harmful to them, and/or reach out for new relationships.

For example, Leticia told us she was very aware of the ways in which binge eating had a negative impact on her relationships, especially before she began treatment with us. It had led her to avoid social activities with her good friends (e.g., canceling at the last minute due to a binge), made her angry at her mother for expecting her to attend family dinners, and played a major role in lowering her self-confidence about meeting new people.

In terms of her relationships with her friends, Leticia said binge eating often caused her to feel ashamed and want to withdraw. When she had made plans, she often ended up canceling if she had had a binge recently, since it made her "feel fat" and she worried that her friends would judge her as she judged herself. Although she felt guilty for being "flaky," she just found it easier to stay home.

Ironically, the few times she didn't cancel were when her mother had family dinner gatherings (see Chaptesr 5 and 6), even though she was quite likely to binge or overeat at these events. Her mother took pride in her cooking and expected the entire family to attend these dinners. Especially since Leticia's father had died, Leticia and her siblings felt responsible for taking care of their mother. Leticia felt guilty about her resentment at being expected to participate and ashamed of her difficulties at the dinners, so she never brought up these issues with her mother.

In terms of forming new relationships, Leticia tended to shy away from opportunities to meet new people, especially in dating situations. Binge eating had lowered her self-confidence, and the relationships she already had seemed hard enough to manage due to her fears of being judged and difficulties expressing her feelings.

EXERCISE 2   Impact of Binge Eating on Your Relationships

a. **How has binge eating interfered with your current relationships?**

_____

_____

_____

_____

_____

_____

Kat wrote:

When I binge eat, I almost always dive into a state of feeling terrible about myself and how I look. This makes me worry that my husband doesn't find me attractive either, which makes me withdraw from him. I can almost literally feel myself recoil when he touches me, which probably makes him feel rejected and less likely to reach out to me. This triggers my insecurities again and leads me to be more likely to binge, starting the cycle again. Ugh!

b. How has binge eating interfered with your ability **to set boundaries in relationships that feel harmful?**

_____

_____

_____

_____

_____

_____

_____

Kat wrote:

Binge eating has always felt like an ugly, shameful secret. My shame and desire to keep my behavior hidden made it hard to feel open and authentic with others. I didn't have access to that part of me that could speak my truth and express my needs. This played out with a "friend" who has betrayed my confidence more than once. I have told her things about myself and my family that I later found she told to others. I am not sure what has kept me from confronting her or breaking off the relationship, but I think it has to do with feeling like I deserve it somehow? Maybe because I betrayed myself with my own behavior for so long by binge eating, it felt almost normal for me to be betrayed by others.

c. How has binge eating interfered with your ability to **form new relation-ships?**

_____

_____

_____

_____

_____

_____

_____

_____

Kat wrote:

Binge eating has taken so much mental energy that my vitality feels like it is lower than it would be otherwise. The energy I do have—the part of me that is interested in meeting new people and learning from them—gets used up in just trying to make it through the day. This is a real loss.

Leticia's plans for attending to her current relationships with her friends included making a decision to accept and follow through on invitations and even to invite others to social events as well. Specifically, during the period before she was supposed to meet with her friends (when she would often cancel at the last minute), her plan was to consult her wise mind. Accessing her wise mind allowed her to remind herself of what she knew deep down to be true—that her friends cared about her, wanted to see her, and did not judge her based on her physical appearance but cared about who she was inside. As she got ready, if she glanced at the mirror, she was to practice dialectical thinking, accepting herself and her behaviors (especially if she had had a binge) *and* her goals for change. She also planned to practice adopting a nonjudgmental stance toward her appearance, which helped her stay calm and stay in touch with her wise mind.

This plan resulted in Leticia having more positive social interactions with her friends and feeling less shame about being unreliable—increasing her overall levels of happiness and self-confidence. These positive emotions, in turn, decreased her vulnerability to binge eating.

Leticia's plan to attend to her relationship with her mother involved first practicing radically accepting her current emotion—in this case her anger and resentment. This meant observing her feelings while adopting a nonjudgmental stance. Acknowledging that her feelings were valid helped her let go of her guilt, helping her access her wise mind, which told her that expressing her feelings to her mother might be a useful strategy.

To Leticia's surprise, when she shared the experience of her difficulty controlling her eating at the dinners, her mother was able to respond in a helpful way. Her mother listened and shared some of her own struggles with eating, and together they came up with a plan in which Leticia's mother decided to serve everyone instead of having the food laid out buffet style. This meant Leticia would no longer have to come face to face with the tempting array of smells and sights of the delicious dishes. Once she shared her feelings with her mother, Leticia's overeating and binge eating at the family dinners decreased markedly and her relationship with her mother felt closer, too.

Leticia's positive experiences with her friends and her mother helped her feel less worried about being judged and more confident that she could express her feelings in new relationships. She decided she was ready to look into online dating, something she had not been willing to do previously. One of her values was to have romance in her life and eventually a family, so it was logical that she had to start somewhere. Her plans to build new relationships included choosing an online dating site and then writing up and placing a profile. As she did so, she planned to practice adopting a nonjudgmental stance and being effective, so that she did not get stuck in negative self-statements nor in trying to write the "perfect" profile. Her wise mind would remind her that any step she took, no matter how small, was a huge step and that she could always edit her profile later.

The simple decision to build new relationships made Leticia feel happier and more hopeful. This led her to take advantage of a free department store clothing consultation she had known was available but had never made use of. Feeling more comfortable and attractive in her clothing helped make getting dressed for social activities less stressful.

EXERCISE 3 Plans to Attend to Relationships

a. Use the space below to **describe your plans to work on your current relationships.**

_____

_____

_____

_____

_____

Kat wrote:

I plan to practice radically accepting my insecurity and anxiety about my attractiveness as something that just is—and something that is certainly more intense if I feel bad about my eating. Hopefully, by accepting that this is how I feel, I will be more able to access my wise mind and share with my husband that I'm not feeling too great and ask him to spend time with me—even though I know a big part of me wants to avoid him. The issue is that when I binge I don't feel attractive. I don't need to put it on him. This should help break the cycle of him feeling rejected if/when I binge.

b. Use the space below to describe your plans to **set boundaries in relationships that feel harmful.**

_____

_____

_____

_____

_____

_____

_____

Kat wrote:

Since starting this program, I have overall really experienced improvements in my binge eating, which has really helped me feel less shame and self-loathing. My wise mind and my desire to live a life that fits more closely with my value of authenticity encourage me to let my friend know how much her betrayals of my confidence have hurt me. I hope she will understand and change so that this doesn't happen anymore. But if she can't empathize or if she gets angry and defensive, I have to wonder if this is the kind of relationship that I want in my life.

c. Use the space below to **describe your plans to form new relationships.**

_____

_____

_____

_____

Kat wrote:

As I write this, I feel more connected to my value of creativity and growth. Not binge eating has allowed my mind to focus on other things, giving me more energy and more courage to seek out events and situations where I can meet people who share my love of singing and the arts in general. I am thinking it would be really fun to go to a weeklong music camp for adults this summer.

Although this program does not focus on improving relationships, we have found that stopping binge eating often ends up doing just this.

Avoid Avoiding

This next skill will also help you change the balance between the number of positive and negative experiences you have by decreasing how often you use avoidance to cope. Many people who binge eat or have other disordered eating behaviors turn to food as a way to avoid dealing with problems or difficulties. They may convince themselves that giving up and binge eating "makes sense" because there is nothing they could effectively do to deal with the problem anyway. Avoiding dealing with problems is similar to capitulating, or convincing yourself that there is absolutely no other choice than to use food in a given situation. When you avoid difficulties by binge eating, you are left not only with the problem itself but also with new problems—the negative consequences of the binge as well as the negative consequences of acting as if you are not capable of dealing directly with difficulties. No one feels very positive when avoiding problem solving or avoiding doing things that are necessary. Feeling greater happiness requires active engagement in your life. Avoidance almost always leads to negative feelings as opposed to feelings of mastery, greater confidence, and control.

The skill of avoiding avoiding involves actively blocking avoidance so you won't turn to binge eating to escape dealing with life's problems. For example, say you are depressed but have a social event you must attend. Your inclination is to want to withdraw or isolate, skipping the event and binge eating at home. Practicing avoiding avoiding would mean actively blocking this urge to skip the event and binge. Instead, you would act opposite to these urges by approaching what you want to avoid and acting in a way that makes you feel competent and confident. The trap that many patients fall into, especially when experiencing emotions like depression, is that they want to feel happier and more motivated before they change their behavior. They say to themselves: "First I want to feel like going out and being with friends, then I'll do it." But the truth is that the most effective treatments for depression work in exactly the opposite way—by having patients get involved in activities first, *before* they feel like it. Their depression then improves. Behavior change leads to mood change, not the other way around. Behaving in ways that are opposite to your emotion communicates a new and different message to your brain. Although these changes do not get processed immediately, they do eventually result in changes in your emotions. When you practice avoiding avoiding and socializing when you are depressed, positive emotional changes eventually take place.

Are you aware of what it is you are trying to avoid when you turn to binge eating? Some of our patients have a lot of awareness, while others are so accustomed to avoiding that they turn to food almost automatically. Therefore, it is important to keep avoiding avoiding in mind, especially when you are first learning this skill. You should be on the lookout for small and seemingly inconsequential problems you avoid dealing with—whether by turning to food or just ignoring the problem (which may set you up to turn to food later). At first dealing with problems head on is clearly more difficult than avoiding problems. However, over time it is always much more effective to deal with the problem.

EXERCISE 4 Avoiding Avoiding

a. Take a moment to consult your wise mind and ask: **"What problems or difficulties in my life am I avoiding, either through binge eating or by just ignoring them?"** Write your answer below.

_____

_____

_____

_____

_____

_____

_____

_____

Kat wrote:

I think that all the examples I wrote about (my husband, my "friend," and not meeting new people) are perfect cases of avoiding. I think the plans to ask my husband to spend time with me (when my urge is to avoid him) and to sign up for a summer music camp (when my urge is to avoid meeting new people) are good ways to practice avoiding avoiding.

In the case of my "friend," I think I need to be more specific than I was. I am remembering how I felt the most recent time one of my good friends, who knows my "friend," let me know that my "friend" had told her something about my relationship to Tom that I had told my "friend" in confidence. When I learned my "friend" had betrayed me again, I felt so hurt and confused and angry—I felt unable to confront her and unable to tolerate how upset I was that I had binged. And after I binged, I felt even less like I deserved to stand up for myself with her.

b. In the space provided (using extra paper if necessary), **write down a plan, or a small action step, to practice avoiding avoiding** so that you act opposite to the urge to avoid.

_____

_____

_____

_____

_____

_____

_____

_____

Kat wrote:

I need to have an honest conversation with my "friend" about the fact that she told others about things that I had told her in confidence. A part of me is so scared and wants to avoid conflict like I always have, but I will act opposite to this urge and will talk with her. What is the worst that can happen? If our friendship ends, I can handle that. What I find so scary is being honest, but I can use my skills of diaphragmatic breathing and wise mind to help me stay calm and centered. I can write out ahead of time the main things I want to say, including that I want to understand why she did this and to be able to build back trust that this won't happen again. I don't have to say everything perfectly.

> *What's important is that I am not avoiding this any longer and am being authentic. Once I've said what I plan to, it will be my turn to lis-ten. Either she will meet me with openness and an apology and we will be able to move past this or she will be angry and defensive and we will not. Either way, I will be OK.*
>
> *I will e-mail her and ask her to go to coffee next week.*

Being Mindful of Positive Emotions

Besides making too little time for positive events, people who binge eat also tend to be "experts" at distracting or undercutting the positive emotions they do have with self-criticism, guilt, and worry. They may find themselves wondering when the positive experience will end or whether they deserve the positive experience, or they may be concerned about how much more might be expected of them because of the positive experience and attention. Such concerns can interfere with your awareness and enjoyment of positive experiences so that you retain only fleeting moments of them.

Being mindful of positive emotions helps your pleasant emotions endure, instead of allowing secondary reactions (e.g., worry, guilt) to "spoil your fun."

Do you experience the problems mentioned above? Perhaps you have enjoyed something and found yourself laughing only to interrupt your enjoyment with a sense of shame, saying to yourself, "I'm being too loud." Or perhaps you have experienced positive emotions such as pride and a sense of accomplishment but have undercut those feelings with a secondary emotion such as guilt by thinking, "I should not feel happy if others are not happy" or "I should not experience pride about my own accomplishments if someone else isn't just as or more successful."

EXERCISE 5 Interrupting Positive Emotions with Guilt, Worry, and Self-Criticism

Do you make time for pleasant events but have a tendency to undercut your enjoyment from these activities by distracting or interrupting yourself with worry, guilt, or self-criticism? Describe below.

_____

_____

_____

_____

_____

_____

_____

_____

_____

Kat wrote:

I was asked to perform at a friend's wedding, which was such a great honor. The day was incredibly beautiful. My friend had her wedding at an old inn in the country—like from a picture book. I sang well, and it felt so good to see her beaming up at me and to know it meant so much to her. For at least a short period I know I felt fully present, but then it felt like too many people came up to me to compliment my singing. One of them asked to contact me to perform again. I was suddenly overcome by anxiety that I wasn't actually that good—that it was just the beautiful setting that was causing people to compliment me. I worried that in another setting I would feel exposed and disappoint them. So instead of continuing to feel good, I just felt anxious.

Practice attending to your positive experience, bringing your full attention to it. If or when you observe that worries or other secondary emotions are intruding, refocus your attention away from the negative and back to your positive emotion for as long as you can. This skill is not about trying to hold on to your positive emotion forever. Instead, the goal is to not destroy, interrupt, or distract yourself from the positive emotions before you have had a chance to fully experience them. Remind yourself that all emotions come and go, both negative and positive ones.

EXERCISE 6 Identifying Positive Emotions You Want to Increase

Think about positive feelings you would like to experience more of, such as pride, joy, and love. Try to identify what secondary reactions might be interfering with getting enjoyment from them. For example, you may be proud of yourself when you finish something at work, but soon after you experience pride you start to judge yourself negatively for not having done a better job. Below, write about the positive experiences you would like to increase and the secondary reactions that may be interfering.

_____

_____

_____

_____

_____

_____

Kat wrote:

I would like to be able to fully appreciate when I sing well. I want to be able to feel proud of myself and not tear myself down with doubts and worries, which are my secondary reactions. I want to experience pride more fully.

The following exercise will help you get the most out of your positive experiences.

EXERCISE 7 Getting the Most Out of Your Positive Experiences

Begin by sitting comfortably in your chair, letting it fully support you. Keep your spine straight, head up, and find a place for your eyes to focus. Take a few deep, flowing breaths in and out. Think of a positive experience you recently had. It can be big or small. While observing that pleasant experience, practice adopting a nonjudgmental stance while focusing on one thing in the moment, allowing yourself to become fully absorbed in the pleasant experience. If you find yourself worrying or having other negative reactions, such as being critical of the experience, gently refocus your attention back on the positive moment, trying to fully participate in it for as long as you can. Write about your experience with this exercise in the space provided.

_____

_____

_____

_____

_____

_____

_____

_____

_____

_____

Kat wrote:

I used this exercise to think about my friend's wedding, when the woman approached me and asked to contact me about performing at another event. I practiced observing how the anxiety started to arise in me as well as the harsh thoughts about how I hadn't really performed that well, it was just the beautiful setting, etc. Instead of reacting to my anxiety or judgmental thoughts, I tried to observe them and practice adopting a nonjudgmental stance by not judging them or myself for having them. I just gently brought my attention back to my friend's happiness and gratitude as she thanked me, which I knew were genuine, and to my pleasure at the lovely day and the lovely setting and how glad I was to have been a part of it.

Here's what John experienced:

John had let his hobbies and some of his friendships drop away since his most recent promotion. Partly because he was always so self-critical, he worried that he didn't really deserve the promotion and demanded even more of himself so his boss would not have any cause to criticize him. So he worked harder. At the end of a long day, he would feel tired and just wanted to "veg." More often than not, especially before starting this program, "vegging" involved binge eating.

As his hobbies and friendships drifted away and his binge eating increased, John's mood worsened and he ended up feeling even more depleted by the evening and on weekends. In some ways he knew getting back into his prior activities, like getting together with friends or spending time sketching, which he enjoyed and was good at, would help. But he kept putting these off.

John appreciated the logic in our discussion of how important it was to balance the number of negative experiences with more positive ones and to enjoy positive experiences more fully when they happened. Thinking of our suggestions as straightforward common sense helped him be more willing to follow through on them because they didn't sound too self-indulgent.

He began by planning daily pleasant events that included even just a few minutes of sketching at his desk while at work. He found that the sketching not only was pleasant but also gave him a sense of mastery. In addition, he practiced a combination of attending to his relationships and avoiding avoiding during the evening when he wanted to "veg." Instead of turning to binge eating and giving in to the urge to isolate, he reached out to talk with friends by telephone or video chat. These conversations, though brief, helped him feel more connected while still allowing him room in his evening to relax. Over time, taking small steps to increase his daily positive activities, attend to his relationships, and avoid avoiding helped him experience more positive emotions, have more energy on weekday evenings and weekends (even signing up for a weekend art class), be more productive at his job, and significantly decrease his binge eating.

Chapter 11 Summary

This chapter discussed two skills you can use to increase the positive emotions you experience, decrease your risk of binge eating, and improve your overall quality of life. The skill of *building positive experiences* addresses the imbalance between positive and negative experiences, and *being mindful of positive emotions* enhances your enjoyment of the positive emotions you do experience.

Four methods were mentioned to help you in building positive experiences. The first involves increasing the number of pleasant activities you engage in on a daily basis, such as gardening or listening to music. The second involves setting long-term goals based on your values in ways that will make your life more satisfying. The third, attending to relationships, involves findings ways to strengthen your existing relationships, set boundaries with harmful relationships, and build new relationships. The final method is to avoid avoiding, or to decrease your use of avoidance, especially when it involves turning to binge eating as a coping mechanism.

The second part of this chapter discussed the skill of being mindful of positive emotions. Some people have a tendency to interrupt their positive experiences with worry, guilt, or self-criticism. By stopping these secondary reactions, you allow yourself to experience greater pleasures from the positive experiences you have.

Both skills can improve your overall mood, make it easier to access your wise mind, and lower the likelihood of binge eating or other problem behaviors.

Homework

Remember to check the box after you have completed each homework assignment.

HOMEWORK EXERCISE 11-A

Planning Pleasant Activities for This Coming Week

Write down pleasant activities you would like to engage in over the next week. Write down one activity for each day. The activity can be the same for multiple days. The important thing is that you are deciding to engage in a pleasant activity each day.

Monday: _____

Tuesday: _____

Wednesday: _____

Thursday: _____

Friday: _____

Saturday: _____

Sunday: _____

❑ I have completed each of these pleasant activities this week.

HOMEWORK EXERCISE 11-B

Worksheet for Increasing Positive Events

Use the worksheet "Increasing Positive Events" on page 214 to set up specific goals in the different areas intended to increase positive emotions, such as by attending to relationships, avoiding avoiding, and building mastery (see Chapter 10). (See the end of the Contents for information on printing out additional copies.) You can also use this sheet to track when you create a positive experience for yourself. Write down a small, specific first step or steps you can take over the next week to work on achieving these goals.

_____

_____

_____

_____

_____

_____

❑ I have filled out the worksheet for increasing positive events and accomplished the first step I wrote down above.

❑ I have filled out my Diary Card daily.

❑ I have filled out at least one Behavioral Chain Analysis Form this week.

❑ I have used the skills I find most helpful so that I can use my wise mind and stop binge eating or other problem behaviors before they happen.

Increasing Positive Events

Increased daily pleasant activities (circle):   M   T   W   Th   F   S   Sun

Describe: _____

_____

_____

_____

Long-term goals worked on:

_____

_____

_____

_____

Attended to relationships (describe):

_____

_____

_____

_____

Avoided avoiding (describe):

_____

_____

_____

_____

Mindfulness of positive experiences that occurred (check which apply):

_____ Focused (and refocused) attention on positive experiences

_____ Did not become distracted from worries about positive experience

12

Distress Tolerance

You've now learned the skills in this program's first two modules: mindfulness and emotion regulation. Many of our patients say they find the skills in the third module, distress tolerance, the most useful of all.

Distress tolerance skills are intended to help you when you're experiencing pain, difficulty, or distress during situations over which you have no control or when you feel so emotionally overloaded that all of your mindfulness and emotion regulation skills have "gone out the window." These are the skills to turn to when your distress level is at such a peak that you simply lack the capacity or willingness to access your wise mind for guidance and apply dialectical thinking, radical acceptance, or other tools from this program. Distress tolerance skills can help you tolerate the emotions of the current moment without making things worse by turning to a destructive behavior like binge eating.

Distress tolerance skills fall into two groups: acceptance skills, which involve helping you let go of struggling with the reality of the situation you are in (though this doesn't necessarily imply you approve of the situation), and crisis survival skills, specific strategies for surviving emergencies. If you're wondering how we define *crisis*, it's not our definition that counts—it's yours. Crisis survival skills can certainly help you cope with life's big challenging or traumatic events and emergencies—accidents, serious illness, the death of a loved one, natural disasters—but also with those unwelcome surprises that might look like "small stuff" to someone else but feel quite distressing to you in the moment, whether it's a delayed or canceled flight, a stolen wallet, a bounced check, a flat tire, or a bad haircut.

Accepting Life as It Is: Radical Acceptance and Half-Smiling

Pain and distress are a part of life. Living skillfully involves accepting that they cannot be avoided entirely. As we've noted before, being able to deal with the reality of difficult events can spare you the extra pain that comes from trying to deny, avoid, or fight your emotional response. Radical acceptance is not a pain-killer; it helps you get through the very natural reaction (pain) to crises and other distress and avoid expanding or extending it by letting it fester while you deny it or distract yourself or do things that make matters worse, like binge eating.

Radical acceptance embodies the spirit of DBT in that you remain aware of the current situation and accept it without evaluating and judging it. You know that this is not easy to do, but at this point in the program you've acquired valuable skills to substitute for the reflexive urge to judge, blame, resist, deny, and run to a temporarily and unsatisfyingly soothing fix like binge eating.

The skills you've learned represent new choices for how you respond to your emotions. The same is true of radical acceptance. When you radically accept your situation, yourself, and your emotions, it is important to realize that you are making a choice. You are *choosing* acceptance. Sometimes difficult situations leave us feeling as if they rob us of choices. But every situation offers a choice—a choice between accepting the situation, dealing with it, and overcoming it, and ignoring or denying the situation and therefore dealing with it ineffectively or destructively (for example, by binge eating). To make the choice of radical acceptance, remember that accepting reality is *acknowledging* reality as it is, not *approving* of it. You can both accept reality and simultaneously not approve of it. This dialectical approach can help you make the often challenging choice of radical acceptance.

Once you have chosen to accept reality as it is, you can do what is necessary in the situation. The next skill, half-smiling, is designed to help with acceptance of difficult situations.

Half-Smiling

This simple skill is deceptively powerful, and many of our patients tell us it becomes one of their favorites. The aim of half-smiling is to help you develop an accepting inner attitude by assuming an outward facial expression of acceptance—the half-smile.

When your facial muscles are tight or your jaw is set, it is very difficult to accept something. The outer tightness is incompatible with an accepting inner attitude. With half-smiling, the muscles of the face are relaxed. So when you use a half-smile—a serene, accepting smile—you are increasing your chances of experiencing internal acceptance.

Experimental evidence shows that the face communicates with the brain. You are probably used to thinking of it the other way around—that you feel an emotion such as sadness or happiness internally, and that internal experience then sends a signal to your face to frown or smile. Yet there is evidence that the feedback also works in the other direction. For example, researchers conducted a study in which participants were given instructions to assume various facial positions or expressions. The instructions to adjust their facial muscles were given slowly and in no clear sequence so that the participants did not know what expression their faces ended up assuming. Interestingly, the researchers found that participants who adopted an angry expression were more likely to experience feelings of anger, and those whose outer expression conveyed sadness were more likely to feel sad, and so on. The researchers concluded that the participants' outward facial expressions triggered their inner emotional experiences—evidence that our bodies communicate with and give feedback to our brains.

We hope that trying the half-smiling exercise will allow you to get a sense of the power of this facial feedback for yourself.

EXERCISE 1 Practicing Half-Smiling

"Begin by putting your face in a neutral position. If it helps you to practice, you can close your eyes, but there is no need to.

"From your neutral face, place your facial muscles in a very angry expression, like one you'd make if you were really infuriated. Push your forehead muscles together in a frown, with your eyebrows turned down in the center. Pull up your upper lip so your teeth show, widen or flare your nostrils, bulge out your eyes, and tense your jaw muscles so that your teeth grind. This is a strong, fierce expression. With your face in this position, take a moment to pay attention to your inner experience. . . .

"Then bring your face back to your neutral expression again, taking several deep breaths from your diaphragm.

"From your neutral face, begin to put your muscles in the expression you'd have if you were really and truly afraid or highly anxious—the face of fear. Widen your eyes, lift your eyebrows and pull them together, stretch out your lips, and pull your lower lip down. With your face in this position, take a moment to pay attention to your inner experience.

"Then once again bring your face back to your neutral facial expression, taking several deep breaths from your diaphragm.

"Next, from your neutral face expression, put your facial muscles into a sad face, maybe even one that is grief stricken or utterly defeated. Let your face droop down, including the lower corners of your mouth, perhaps making your lower lip shake or tremble. Draw your eyebrows together and place your forehead muscles into a frown. With your face in this position, take a moment to pay attention to your inner experience.

"Next, try a half-smile. It is important to remember that when you half-smile, your face is completely relaxed. It can help to imagine a cool iron, or the cool and skillful hands of a masseuse, smoothing the muscles on your face and neck. Your muscles are just 'hanging' on your face, with the iron or the masseuse's gentle fingers smoothing over your forehead, temples, cheek-bones, chin, neck, and shoulders.

"Then, ever so slightly, turn the corners of your lips up toward your ears. It's just a slight upturn of the lips, not really a smile, but it's still perceptibly different from the neutral face. This upward turn of the lips is not a tense expression—it's not a grin or a smirk. Perhaps it might help to think of the Mona Lisa smile.

"Let yourself take several moments, breathing in and out from your dia-phragm, to pay attention to your internal experience while you maintain your half-smile."

What did you notice about your inner experience when you adopted the differ-ent facial expressions and then finally the half-smile? With the half-smile, did you notice a greater openness to acceptance? Write about your experience below.

_____

_____

_____

_____

_____

_____

_____

Kat wrote:

I noticed that when I contorted my face into the angry, scared, or sad expressions, the muscles in my entire body became tense. I felt a pit of stress in my stomach, and my heart started beating faster. When I changed to the half-smile, with the upturn of my lips, I felt calmer. I felt a bubble of something, maybe even happiness, come up inside me. I can see how feeling more peaceful would allow me to feel more accepting.

Practicing the half-smile is not intended to mask, deny, or hide your emo-tions. Choosing to half-smile involves an acknowledgment of the situation you are facing, followed by choosing to help facilitate your inner acceptance of this reality through changing your external facial expression. You are making a decision to change your emotional state by changing the feedback your brain receives from your facial muscles. Compared to some of the other skills we have taught, which involve changing how you think about your experience, half-smiling is a physical behavior, like diaphragmatic breathing, that can alter your internal experience.

While half-smiling is an extremely useful skill, it may not be helpful during moments when you feel unable or unwilling to accept the situation you find yourself in—when you cannot locate your wise mind or feel that you would not want to listen to it, even if you could. This is where the crisis survival skills come in.

Crisis Survival Skills

As noted above, the crisis survival skills are skills for tolerating painful events and emotions when it feels like your skills have "gone out the window." The emphasis here is on getting through the periods of crisis or emergency effectively, or at least not making matters worse, when you cannot make things better right away. The crisis survival skills are not designed to solve underlying issues or change the situation. But by getting temporary relief, you can shore yourself up so that you can respond effectively when there is an opportunity to do so. Remember while practicing a crisis survival skill to also use the skill of focusing on one thing in the moment. The crisis survival skills will not be as effective at giving you temporary relief if you use them while simultaneously continuing to be preoccupied with the crisis.

Surviving a crisis without making matters worse takes a great deal of effort, especially at first. In the past, when you felt pushed beyond your emotional limits, binge eating was likely your old "tried-and-true" or "go-to" behavior. It might be difficult to believe anything else could really "work." Later in this chapter we discuss how Angela struggled with this belief. While binge eating is temporarily effective and perhaps was the best option you had for coping with emotions that felt unmanageable, the reason you committed to stop binge eating in Chapter 2 was that you recognized past crises in your life were never solved but instead were made worse by binge eating. At best, binge eating may have temporarily "worked" by removing you from a crisis.

The crisis survival skills offer you that chance to take a break and develop a new perspective without having to pay the destructive longer-term costs of binge eating.

Remember before you start on these skills that what is a crisis is subjective. What one person might not find so distressing could be extremely distressing to another to the point of triggering a binge. But we recommend that you use the crisis survival skills for everyday crises rather than keeping them in reserve for only the big crises. One definition of a crisis might be: a situation during which one feels overwhelmed and helpless. While some people lose interest in food entirely during such situations, binge eaters often find themselves more preoccupied with food because it helps them numb, avoid, or escape their distress. The crisis survival skills offer you a much more effective way to take a needed break. Later, when you are feeling less overwhelmed, you can decide what other skills to use or other actions (if any) to take.

The crisis survival skills include distraction skills, self-soothing skills, and thinking of the pros and cons of tolerating your distress. These diverse crisis survival skills have been developed because crisis situations vary and require the use of different skills. It is important to maintain an open mind while practicing these skills. You may have to experiment to find the skill that is most effective in a particular crisis.

EXERCISE 2   Your Current Crises

In the space provided, **write about the situations you need to "survive" in your life right now**—situations that you cannot make better, at least in this moment.

_____

_____

_____

_____

_____

_____

_____

_____

Kat wrote:

The true crisis in my life right now is my friend's diagnosis with dementia. But somehow there are smaller things that end up feeling very intense. Like last week I tried a new hair stylist, and she cut off 3 more inches of my hair than I had asked, just as I had a big singing performance coming up. Also, my husband is going away on a business trip just as we have to file the extension on our tax return, leaving me with what feels like all the work. These things feel so overwhelming that I'm having strong urges to binge.

Distraction Skills

The purpose of distraction skills is to temporarily remove yourself from emotional triggers or situations that are too overwhelming. At such times you need to refocus outside of yourself and outside of the situation to give yourself a needed break. The distraction skills are not intended as a means of avoiding or denying reality to pretend there isn't a crisis. The idea is to use the distraction skills to interrupt the crisis long enough to reduce your tension so that when you return to dealing with the crisis you're at least a little bit renewed or have a slightly different perspective on things. Ideally you'd be able to use your mindfulness or emotion regulation skills to cope with whatever situation you find yourself in. However, sometimes you need a little break before you are able to do so.

Examples of different ways to practice the distraction skills are described below and summarized in the box on page 222.

ACTIVITIES

One way to distract is with *activities*. These activities, especially when done mindfully, can occupy and distract you so that your urges to binge or engage in other destructive behaviors are reduced. Examples include exercise, hobbies, cleaning, going to events, calling/texting, visiting with a friend, and doing a puzzle.

CONTRIBUTING

Another means of practicing distracting is by *contributing*. By contributing you get in touch with a different experience than that of the current crisis. Many of our patients report this to be very useful. The contribution does not have to be a big one—it might simply be saying hello to someone. Other examples of contributing include helping a neighbor with a chore, doing something extra or kind for a family member or friend, or anything else that allows you to contribute positively to someone else's life.

COMPARISONS

Another type of distraction involves making *comparisons*. It can be helpful to think of others who are experiencing a worse situation or who are less fortunate. This might initially sound odd or even depressing, but we encourage you to try it.

OPPOSITE EMOTIONS

Bringing up *opposite emotions* is another type of distraction. By becoming involved in something that will create a different emotion from the upsetting one that you are experiencing in the crisis, you are distracting yourself with an opposite feeling. Distracting with positive emotions is often particularly helpful. Some suggestions include watching comedies (movies or TV shows), listening to music,

Crisis Survival: Distraction Skills

Distract using

Activities, such as:

- Exercise
- Hobbies
- Cleaning
- Going to events
- Calling/texting or visiting a friend
- Doing a puzzle

Contributing, such as:

- Simply saying hello to someone
- Helping a neighbor or friend with a chore
- Doing something kind for a family member or friend
- Volunteering to help with a project
- Making an online donation
- Reaching out to stay in touch with an elderly relative

Comparisons, such as:

- Thinking of others experiencing a worse situation or who are less fortunate

Opposite emotions, such as:

- Watching comedies (movies or TV shows)
- Listening to music
- Reading a funny book

Pushing away, such as:

- Physically removing yourself from the situation (taking a bathroom break, taking a short walk)
- Leaving mentally, if you cannot leave physically, perhaps by envisioning boxing up the overwhelming situation or feelings and putting them high on a shelf

Other intense sensations that help you experience something different, such as:

- Standing under a hot shower
- Immersing your face in ice water
- Holding ice cubes in your hands
- Listening to very loud music

reading a funny book—anything that will get you involved in a different emotional experience.

PUSHING AWAY

You can also distract through *pushing away*. Sometimes physically removing yourself can be quite helpful. If you cannot leave physically, you can leave mentally—perhaps by envisioning boxing up the overwhelming situation or feelings and sending them off or putting them high on a shelf. Again the purpose of this skill is to help you have a temporary break.

OTHER INTENSE SENSATIONS

Another type of distraction involves making use of *other intense sensations*. You might stand under a really hot shower, immerse your face in ice water (many find this particularly effective for creating a calming response), hold ice cubes in your hands, listen to very loud music, and so on. We encourage you to do things that distract you from whatever the emotional trigger is so that you can experience something different.

EXERCISE 3 Using the Distraction Skills

Which of the distraction skills mentioned so far seem like they **would be helpful to try?** Describe them in the space provided.

_____

_____

_____

_____

_____

_____

Kat wrote:

When I am overwhelmed by my anger at my husband for abandoning me to work on the tax situation and I can no longer focus, I will use pushing away and take a short walk. Maybe I will also try other intense sensations like taking a really hot shower.

Self-Soothing Skills

Do you have a tendency to ignore your body's sensations when in a crisis?

Yes   No

Would skills designed to help you be gentle with yourself be useful for everyday crises as well as for especially difficult times?

Yes   No

When you are emotionally overwhelmed, finding ways to comfort and nurture yourself can be very effective. While being compassionate and gentle to yourself is likely something you would suggest to someone else in a crisis, we have a feeling that when *you're* in a crisis, the idea of being kind to yourself probably does not come to mind. In fact, perhaps you criticize yourself for experiencing the crisis and for not being able to resolve it. Having compassion for yourself, however, is more effective.

Turning to find comfort (or distraction, numbing, escape) in food may feel kind in the moment. However, your wise mind knows and your own experience has shown you that this behavior is ultimately an extremely damaging way to cope—harmful to your self-esteem, your body, your relationships with others, and your relationship with yourself. That is why you are using this program and increasing your list of effective coping strategies, for example, with self-soothing skills.

The self-soothing skills can be organized by the five senses. Specifically, self-soothing involves filling one or all of your senses with pleasant experiences. These skills are described below and summarized in the box on the facing page.

To practice self-soothing with *vision*, you might buy a beautiful flower, light a candle, visit a museum filled with beautiful art, immerse yourself in nature, and/or go out in the middle of the night to look at the stars. When practicing this skill, you should try to be mindful of each sight that passes in front of you. You can use some of the mindfulness skills you have already learned—such as observing, focusing on one thing in the moment, and adopting a nonjudgmental stance. By putting yourself in an accepting state of mind in just this one moment, you may find it easier to get through a crisis without making it worse.

When you practice self-soothing with *hearing*, you might try listening to beautiful, peaceful music. Or practice paying attention to the sounds of nature around you, such as the chirping of birds or other wildlife. Another idea would be to hum a soothing song to yourself.

Self-soothing can also involve the sense of *smell*. You might apply your favorite perfume or lotions, light a scented candle, boil cinnamon, and/or mindfully breathe in the fresh smells of nature.

Self-Soothing with the Five Senses

Vision

- Buy a beautiful flower.
- Light a candle.
- Visit a museum filled with beautiful art.
- Go out in nature.
- Watch the stars.

Hearing

- Listen to beautiful, peaceful music.
- Pay attention to the sounds of nature around you, such as the chirping of birds or other wildlife.
- Hum a soothing song to yourself.

Smell

- Apply your favorite perfume or lotions.
- Light a scented candle.
- Boil cinnamon.
- Mindfully breathe in the fresh smells of nature.

Taste (remember to consult your wise mind first)

- Have a soothing drink, like hot tea or decaffeinated coffee.
- Mindfully suck on a piece of sugar-free candy.

Touch

- Take a bubble bath.
- Have a massage.
- Get a manicure or pedicure.
- Pet a dog or cat.
- Soak your feet.
- Put a cold compress on your forehead.
- Cuddle with a plush toy or under a soft or heated blanket.

Self-soothing with *taste* may or may not work well for you. If you decide to practice it, you will need to use your wise mind. One suggestion is to have a soothing drink—like a cup of hot tea or decaffeinated coffee, or to mindfully suck on a piece of sugar-free candy. If you are emotionally vulnerable, it is vital to use only foods that will *not* trigger you to binge. Many people are able to self-soothe with food in ways that are not harmful. The key is eating mindfully and with awareness.

When self-soothing with *touch*, you could take a bubble bath, have a massage, treat yourself to a manicure or pedicure, pet your dog or cat, soak your feet, put a cold compress on your forehead, or cuddle with a plush toy or under a soft or heated blanket.

You may be wondering how you can make sure you use crisis survival skills when you need them. The following experiential exercise will help you practice so that you will be more likely to access the crisis survival skills when a crisis occurs.

EXERCISE 4 Using Self-Soothing Skills

Which of the self-soothing skills mentioned seem like they would be helpful to try? Describe in the space provided.

_____

_____

_____

_____

_____

_____

Kat wrote:

I love all of these. I already use many of them—I have my animals that I pet on my lap and I enjoy listening to music as a way to self-soothe. I think that I will treat myself to a beautiful tea set that I've been admiring at a local second-hand store. It's not too expensive, but it's lovely and will make enjoying tea that much more special. I am going to download some nature sounds of rainwater because I find that really soothing and I want to have that for times when I am stuck in traffic. Sort of a self-soothing "on the go." I would also like to take time, especially when I am overwhelmed, to go into my backyard and look up at the clouds during the day or the stars at night—even if for just a moment.

The last crisis survival skill that will be discussed is called thinking of pros and cons.

Thinking of Pros and Cons

The skill of thinking of pros and cons gives you a chance to think, in a very deliberate way, of the advantages and disadvantages of tolerating your current distress in an effective, nondestructive way. The straightforward observation of the facts can be extremely useful in helping you make practical decisions when you are feeling emotionally overwhelmed during a crisis.

The best way to learn about this skill is to practice it. In the following experiential exercise, we will ask you to consider the pros and cons of your various options for tolerating distress in the middle of a crisis. After you have done so, we think you will better understand its usefulness.

EXERCISE 5 Practicing Thinking of Pros and Cons

Take a moment to think about what constitutes a crisis for you, the kind of situation in which, at least in the past, you turned to binge eating. Remember that the definition of a crisis is a personal one. Perhaps a crisis was facing the pressures of work or school deadlines you felt you couldn't meet. Or an argument with a friend or loved one, the kind of argument you felt had damaged the relationship to the point where it might not recover. Or perhaps a crisis was finding a parking ticket you had forgotten to pay on time, so now you had to add a hefty fine. For this exercise, picture a crisis in which you are experiencing strong urges to binge. This crisis could be from the past, one you are currently facing, or one you'd be very worried would tempt you in the future.

Imagine you are currently right in the middle of this crisis. Briefly describe the situation in the space provided.

_____

_____

_____

_____

Kat wrote:

What's causing me to want to binge is having gotten a bad haircut before the gig. I feel embarrassed that I look terrible and angry at myself for having tried a new stylist in the first place. I also feel embarrassed that I care

*since I know it shouldn't matter—which makes me want to binge, too. I'm
ashamed of myself for wanting to cancel and not show up.*

a. **Tolerating distress using effective coping skills: PROS.** The first step
   is to think about the PROS, or positive consequences, of TOLERATING
   your distress by using effective, healthy coping skills. These pros might
   include how good you will feel if you don't act impulsively in this moment or
   the self-respect you will feel as you make progress toward your long-term
   goals rather than repeating old patterns and feeling you are backsliding,
   which makes you feel ashamed and comes at a high cost.

   In the space provided, write the **PROS or advantages of tolerating
   your distress** in an effective way.

   1. _____

   _____

   _____

   2. _____

   _____

   _____

   3. _____

   _____

   _____

   4. _____

   _____

   _____

Kat wrote:

1. *I will feel greater self-respect by tolerating my embarrassment and
   anger over my haircut rather than having a binge. Living by my
   values of self-acceptance will help me feel compassion, dignity, and a
   sense of grace.*

2. *I will not experience the guilt and shame I always get after I binge—
   which will help me be more comfortable with my appearance instead
   of making things worse.*

3. *Binge eating will only make it easier for me to avoid showing up for
   the performance (I'm in a group, and while I need to be there, I don't
   do solos). By being a professional and acting opposite of the urge to*

avoid I will feel good about breaking my bad pattern of avoiding things that make me anxious.

4. *I value growth, and by not binge eating I can honestly tell myself that I would be taking positive steps toward living authentically.*

b. **Tolerating distress using effective coping skills: CONS.** Now think about the CONS, or negative consequences, of TOLERATING your distress in an effective way. That is, what are the negative consequences of using effective coping skills to tolerate distress?

In the space below discuss the **CONS or disadvantages of not turning to a destructive behavior,** such as binge eating. If you're finding it hard to come up with many CONS, that's OK!

1. _____

_____

_____

2. _____

_____

_____

3. _____

_____

_____

4. _____

_____

_____

Kat wrote:

1. *I will have to truly feel the anxiety of performing when I know or at least believe my hair looks ridiculous.*

2. *I won't have the immediate relief from canceling my performance.*

3. *I won't have the temporary feeling of control and escape by indulging in whatever I feel like eating.*

c. **Choosing to not tolerate your distress by using ineffective, unhealthy coping skills: PROS.** Now think about the PROS of NOT TOLERATING your distress, and instead using an ultimately ineffective coping skill like binge eating. The question to ask yourself is "What are the advantages of allowing myself to act impulsively and binge eat?" We do not doubt that you, like many of our patients, may have experienced quite real, though temporary, benefits in the past when you used food to avoid the pain of the current moment. Binge eating can work briefly to manage painful feelings and to allow you to numb out or avoid them.

In the space below discuss the **PROS of choosing to not tolerate your distress by turning to binge eating.**

1. _____

_____

_____

2. _____

_____

_____

3. _____

_____

_____

4. _____

_____

_____

Kat wrote:

1. *I get to escape feeling anxious and upset about the way I look.*

2. *I get to instantly take care of my anger at myself for trying a new stylist right before a big performance by distracting myself with food.*

3. *I get to feel in control and do whatever I want in a situation where the control has been taken away from me.*

d. **Not tolerating distress using ineffective coping skills: CONS.** Finally, think about the CONS, or disadvantages, of NOT TOLERATING your distress and using an ineffective coping skill such as binge eating. What has acting impulsively and misusing food cost you in the past? What would it cost currently—or in the near future—in terms of your self-confidence, mood, relationships, physical well-being, overall quality of life? For example, does binge eating lead to regret, severe self-recrimination, hopelessness, demoralization, depression, feeling physically sick?

In the space below, discuss in a straightforward way the **CONS of choosing to not tolerate your distress by turning to binge eating.**

1. _____
_____
_____

2. _____
_____
_____

3. _____
_____
_____

4. _____
_____
_____

Kat wrote:

1. I will feel tremendous regret, guilt, and shame.

2. I will no doubt judge myself for sabotaging the progress I have made.

3. I will feel incompetent and unable to cope with one of life's everyday challenges.

4. My regret, guilt, and shame will probably trigger urges to binge again. I always tell myself that it will be "just this once" but the truth is that each binge makes me more vulnerable to another one.

e. **Comparing the PROS and CONS.** The last step is to compare your PROS and CONS responses. Please do so in the space provided.

_____
_____
_____
_____
_____

Kat wrote:

I found this to be useful. I found that the pros for using effective coping were long-lasting and didn't just address the distress of the moment. It

> *was much easier to think of the cons of giving in to my distress rather than the pros of giving in to my distress.*

Our patients typically find that they have somewhat similar numbers of pros for using ineffective (c: PROS of Binge Eating) and effective (a: PROS of Not Binge Eating) coping skills, but there are usually many more cons to using unhealthy coping skills (d) than healthy coping skills (b).

We hope this exercise helps demonstrate how this skill can be very useful to you in a crisis. One important reason for its effectiveness is that it temporarily removes you from the crisis situation by forcing you to think about the pros and the cons of your behaviors. In addition, it gives you the opportunity to make a truly informed choice about using an effective, healthy coping skill or an ineffective, unhealthy coping skill. As we have stated before, one important way to prevent binge eating is to change how you think of binge eating—from an automatic response to a *choice*. This exercise allows you to do that.

As you try out and use the different coping skills in this chapter, it will be useful to note which ones work best for you. You can write those skills down on a card to keep with you—as we suggest in the homework for this chapter. That way, when you experience an intense emotion you only have to look at the card to review the skills you can use.

As you work on the crisis survival skills, remember that it will take time and practice for you to find them as "helpful" as you found binge eating to be in the past when you felt truly overwhelmed. Don't forget that you were "practicing" binge eating as a coping tool for many years and it will take practice to get the most out of these new coping skills you are learning. We have seen how effective these strategies can be when our patients become used to turning to them instead of binge eating. This was Angela's experience with the distress tolerance skills.

Angela was uncertain about how useful the distress tolerance skills would be. She told us that especially the self-soothing ones sounded somewhat unrealistic and "woo-woo."

"They remind me of advice I always have heard, like take a bubble bath with candles when you're stressed. But am I really going to light candles and have a bubble bath instead of bingeing? The sad truth is that I can't see myself using these skills when I'm at my wit's end, and feeling the kind of awful way I do, like at work sometimes or when I'm upset at home with my husband and we're totally not getting along. It feels like I need and deserve cookies for being willing to stick with how hard life can feel. They seem to help me survive those hard times, even though I always regret binge eating so much. But I can't imagine anything else working when it's really a crisis." Although she had not had a binge in quite some time and felt committed to stopping binge eating, she admitted that on some level she was keeping binge eating in her "back pocket" for emergencies. She worried that when it came down to it, nothing else could be powerful enough to soothe her the way food could when life's pain felt like too much to bear.

We asked Angela to just practice using the distress tolerance skills to help with the small crises in her life and not to worry yet about the big ones. She decided that what binge eating seemed to offer her most was temporary soothing and escape, and so she began to carry lavender-scented hand lotion with her and keep other scented lotions (e.g., lemon, grapefruit) at various places in her home as well as on her desk at work. She used these for difficult times such as mornings when her children resisted waking up for school on time, before and after meetings at work (particularly involving her boss), and so on.

Angela was pleased to see that her distress levels really did drop after she used the lotion. She started branching out and using other types of self-soothing, including buying herself a very soft and huggable plush animal and an adult coloring book. She began using half-smiling as well, particularly when she had to wait on long lines in grocery or department stores.

However, she was embarrassed to admit to us that she still thought of binge eating as her true backup strategy. At least until one day when so many things piled up that it seemed like more than she could handle.

Angela awoke that day feeling cranky from having stayed up late with her daughter to help her complete an assignment for school. Then, at work, she received harsh criticism from her boss on a report, which left her feeling demoralized. Later that day she heard from a friend that a mutual acquaintance, one Angela had always been envious of, had been promoted. By the end of the day, Angela couldn't wait to leave the office and have the day be over. However, her car wouldn't start. She returned to her desk and called emergency roadside assistance, only to find out that, due to high demand, help wasn't available for 1½–2 hours. She texted her husband to let him know. He called back, asking in an irritated voice whether she remembered he had a work event that evening and if she had been taking their car in for regular maintenance. After she admitted she had been late servicing the car, he angrily said that he would change his plans and take care of the kids but would she please take the car in more regularly in the future? Angela felt angry too, both at her husband and at herself. After hanging up, she felt stunned and overwhelmed. Angela suddenly started to think about the chocolates that a coworker always kept in a big glass bowl on her desk. Angela hadn't eaten them for soooo long. She deserved to eat them; this was just too much.

Angela doesn't remember exactly how, but somehow her eyes happened to fall on the large tube of honeysuckle lotion she kept on her desk. Without giving it much thought, it occurred to her to put some on. She didn't think it would stop her from binge eating the chocolate, but as she was rubbing it in, she noticed that she was feeling a little calmer. As she focused on the smell of the lotion and the sensation of it on her hands and arms, she started to think that maybe things weren't so awful and that she wasn't as awful a person as she had been feeling she was. She began to feel the presence of her wise mind and had the thought that it was possible to get through even this situation without a binge—a situation that would certainly have led to binge eating in the past. She imagined how much better she would feel the next day if she didn't feel "hung over" from binge eating. And she knew that if she did start binge eating, she would continue when she got home, likely distancing herself from her husband and children.

She kept massaging the lotion into her hands and thought of ways she could spend the next 2 hours that, instead of the temporary comfort of binge eating, would be comforting but not destructive—like reading a book on her Kindle while listening to some music. She had some healthy snacks in her office that could tide her over, and while eating them she could practice mindful eating. She decided to first call her husband, saying she wanted his help to figure out an appropriate maintenance schedule for her car. He apologized for being so irritated, saying it was just hard for him to make last-minute changes. She felt closer to him and let him know about some of the difficult parts of her day, appreciating his sympathy. The 2 hours passed quickly without binge eating. She was able to make it through without binge eating that evening either and got to sleep early.

Chapter 12 Summary

This chapter discussed several different skills you can use to survive a crisis. Crises can be either large or small, but they are times when the emotion you are feeling may be too intense for you to use the other skills we have discussed in earlier chapters. Radical acceptance was the first skill that was discussed in this chapter. Radical acceptance involves coming to terms with your current situation, deciding to change what you can, and deciding to accept what you cannot change. Acceptance of your current situation may bring enough calm for you to be able to use some of the other skills, such as mindfulness of your current emotion. One skill that can help with radical acceptance is half-smiling. Half-smiling was introduced as a way to change your outward expression, which can influence your internal acceptance.

In addition to radical acceptance three specific kinds of crisis survival skills were discussed. Each is designed to help get you through a crisis so that you can make the best decisions for your overall well-being.

The first crisis survival skill discussed was distraction. Distraction is designed to provide you with temporary relief so that you can get a brief break, recharge your battery, and in the end respond to the situation by being effective. One example discussed was bringing up an emotion opposite to your current emotion.

The second crisis survival skill discussed was self-soothing. Self-soothing is about being gentle and compassionate to yourself during a crisis. Self-soothing involves providing pleasant experiences to one or all of your five senses. One example was using your sense of smell by applying a favorite perfume or lotion.

The last skill discussed was thinking of pros and cons. This involves thinking about the pros and cons of using healthy coping skills, like those in this program, versus unhealthy, ineffective coping skills, like binge eating.

By regularly using all the skills in this program, and by using the distress tolerance skills during crises, you may find that you now have all the necessary skills you need to overcome binge eating.

Homework

Remember to check the box after you have completed each homework assignment.

HOMEWORK EXERCISE 12-A
Practicing Half-Smiling

Practice half-smiling each day for a week. Write about your experiences below.

_____

_____

_____

_____

_____

_____

❏ I have practiced half-smiling once each day this week.

❏ I have written about my experience above.

HOMEWORK EXERCISE 12-B

Practicing Thinking of Pros and Cons

At least one day this week, practice the thinking of pros and cons exercise. If you don't have a situation where this skill would work you can think of a past experience instead.

❑ I have practiced the thinking of pros and cons exercise this week.

HOMEWORK EXERCISE 12-C

Practicing Crisis Survival Skills

During the upcoming week, practice at least three different crisis survival skills each day to become familiar with all of them. It is helpful to track how effective the different crisis survival skills are so that eventually you will have an idea of which ones are most helpful. This includes keeping notes of which category of skills were used (e.g., distracting, self-soothing, thinking of pros and cons), which specific skill was tried (e.g., taking a bubble bath, under self-soothing with touch), and the distress experienced before (from 0 to 100) and after (from 0 to 100). Here is an example of the format you could use:

Day/date:	Crisis survival skill tried	Distress before (0–100)	Distress after (0–100)
_____	_____	_____	_____
_____	_____	_____	_____
_____	_____	_____	_____
_____	_____	_____	_____
_____	_____	_____	_____
_____	_____	_____	_____
_____	_____	_____	_____

❑ I have tried at least three different crisis survival skills each day this week.

HOMEWORK EXERCISE 12-D

Card Listing Most Effective Crisis Survival Skills

Write down on a 3" × 5" card or other piece of paper you can fold and keep with you which specific crisis survival skills were most effective. This way, when you experience an intense emotion, you can pull out the card as a reminder of what skills you can use. You may also want to keep a list on your smartphone.

❏ I have filled out a card with the crisis survival skills I found most effective.

HOMEWORK EXERCISE 12-E

Continuing to Reduce Vulnerability to Emotion Mind

Thinking back to Chapter 10, we would like you to record what specific changes you have made these past weeks to continue to reduce your vulnerability to emotion mind and to binge eating.

_____

_____

_____

_____

_____

_____

❏ I have recorded the changes I have made to continue to reduce my vulnerability to emotion mind and to binge eating.

❏ I have filled out my Diary Card daily.

❏ I have filled out at least one Behavioral Chain Analysis Form this week.

❏ I have used the skills I find most helpful so that I can use my wise mind and stop binge eating or any other problem behaviors before they happen.

13

Reviewing, Planning
for the Future,
and Preventing Relapse

As you are no doubt aware, this book has only so many pages, and you are now coming to the end of them. However, unlike traditional therapist-led therapy, this doesn't mean that your "treatment" is over! This DBT self-help program, including all the skills it has taught you to stop binge eating, will always be here for you. It is *your* program. We hope you will continue to refer to it.

The key to keeping your binge eating under control is to continue to practice the skills so often that you turn to them automatically, the way you once turned automatically to food. As with any discipline, like playing tennis or playing the piano, it's essential to continue to practice to keep up your abilities. Rather than treating this program as a book that you put away on a shelf once you've finished reading it, treat it as a refresher course you'll come back to whenever you need a skills "tune-up."

So that you can get the most out of everything you've learned and continue to use it to your greatest benefit, this chapter provides:

1. A brief review of this program's approach and the skills taught (focusing on those you found most helpful)

2. A review of your progress to date and any remaining binge eating

3. Advice on planning for the future, including coping ahead, one final skill to help you prevent a relapse in case you find yourself slipping or experiencing urges to slip

4. Guidance on identifying any barriers that interfere with your continuing to build a satisfying and rewarding quality of life

A Brief Review of the Program

- We began this program by explaining what caused binge eating and why, despite the pain it caused you, you still had so much trouble stopping.

- Understanding these explanations is the key to avoiding becoming stuck in unhelpful self-judgment. It is therefore important to make sure that the points in this brief review sound familiar.

- As described in Chapter 1, when emotions feel too intense to be tolerated, binge eating "works" by temporarily allowing you to avoid, numb, escape, distract, and/or self-soothe.

- What makes binge eaters find intense emotions difficult to tolerate, compared to non-binge-eaters, involves both *biological* and *environmental/social* components.

- Biologically speaking, you are likely to be emotionally sensitive or to be "thinner skinned." It takes less to provoke an emotional reaction in you than in others, your emotional reactions are likely more intense, and your recovery time after an emotional reaction is longer.

- You are more likely to find food appealing even when you're not physically hungry, compared to others—especially when you're feeling emotionally distressed.

- Environmentally/socially speaking, as you were growing up and/or as an adult you likely were told (directly or indirectly) that your feelings or reactions were "wrong" or invalid. Lacking emotional attunement, you learned to invalidate your own emotional reactions to the point that perhaps you regularly ignored, suppressed, and no longer even recognized your emotional responses.

- Over time, this mismatch between your biological vulnerability and environmental invalidation led you to have increasing difficulty tolerating intense emotions, increasing the likelihood of bingeing to escape, numb, or avoid emotional distress, at least temporarily.

- This program offers you an alternative to binge eating by teaching you skills and strategies for coping with emotional distress. The skills teach you how to cope with intense emotions so that you feel less compelled, in the moment, to turn to food.

- Binge eating was a behavior you had learned, and the good news was you could *un*learn it.

Skills Review

By this point in the program, we know that you likely have your favorite skills. We want to take this opportunity to remind you that different phases of life, relationships, jobs, housing situations, and so on may call for you to use skills that, when we first presented them, did not seem as compelling as they might seem now or will in the future. That is why we recommend taking the time to review all the skills you have available to you. Starting on the facing page, you'll find a checklist of all the skills taught in this program. You can review it before you do Exercises 1 and 2, checking off whether you've been using each of the skills.

EXERCISE 1 Skills You Currently Find Especially Helpful

List below the 5 to 10 **skills** you have found **especially helpful.** Feel free to add more on a separate page. If you'd like a review, refer to the list of skills on pages 241–244 if needed.

1. _____

2. _____

3. _____

4. _____

5. _____

6. _____

7. _____

8. _____

9. _____

10. _____

Kat wrote:

1. Adopting a Nonjudgmental Stance

2. Wise Mind

3. Diaphragmatic Breathing

4. Crisis Survival Skills—Self-Soothing

5. Mindful Eating

Renewing Your Commitment (Chapter 2): This skill involves renewing as often as possible the formal commitment to stop binge eating that you made in Chapter 2.

❑ Are you beginning your day by rereading the cards you made of the pros of stopping binge eating and the cons of continuing to binge eat?

Wise Mind (Chapter 3): This skill involves getting in touch with a very deep and centered part of yourself, in which your emotions and your rational responses are integrated. In wise mind, you are operating from your best self, and your decisions and actions are in line with your values.

❑ Do you practice accessing your wise mind as often as possible to break links that might lead to binge eating?

Diaphragmatic Breathing (Chapter 3): The skill of diaphragmatic breathing involves practicing deep breathing and focusing on your breath. This type of breathing lowers stress and can facilitate mindfulness, or your awareness of being "here and now," in the present moment.

❑ Are you practicing diaphragmatic breathing when you are experiencing the urge to binge eat, a preoccupation with food, emotional discomfort, and/or physical tension?

Dialectical Thinking (Chapter 5): The skill of dialectal thinking involves being able to think flexibly instead of getting stuck in emotion mind and its rigid, perfectionistic, "black-and-white" mindset.

❑ Are you practicing using dialectical thinking and the Olympic athlete metaphor so that you don't have to abandon your important goal of stopping binge eating, despite not always achieving it?

❑ Are you also thinking dialectically to help yourself accept conflicting feelings about giving up binge eating as well as accepting yourself exactly as you are right now *and* committing to change?

Observing (Chapter 5): The skill of observing offers you the opportunity to experience physical sensations as well as intense emotions without getting caught up in, judging, or reacting to them.

❑ Are you using observing to help you become unstuck from your emotion mind and make it easier to access your wise mind?

Adopting a Nonjudgmental Stance (Chapter 6): This skill involves not judging yourself or your emotions or behaviors in moral terms—such as good or bad, right or wrong, worthwhile or worthless. Are you practicing adopting a nonjudgmental stance toward yourself?

(continued)

❑ For example, instead of making judgmental self-statements like "I'm a failure" or "I shouldn't be feeling this way—I'm a terrible person," are you practicing observing just the facts, remembering that you can accept how you feel without necessarily approving of it or acting on it?

❑ Are you adopting a nonjudgmental stance to help you move from emotion mind to wise mind to avoid binge eating?

Focusing on One Thing in the Moment (Chapter 6): This skill involves not multitasking but instead placing your entire focus or attention on one thing, for one moment at a time.

❑ Are you practicing focusing on one thing in the moment on a regular basis to help you direct your attention without letting your mind wander to something else?

❑ Have you been getting the most you can from this skill by taking opportunities to give yourself a break and slow down so that you can access your wise mind to help you deal with urges to binge eat?

Being Effective (Chapter 6): This skill means giving up being right, correct, perfect, and/or the view that things must be exactly as you want them to be. Instead, being effective means doing what is needed to reach your goals. In some cases you *may* be right and your way *may* be the fair way, but being effective requires accepting the realities of the situation you are in during that moment.

❑ Are you practicing being effective to stop binge eating and get the most out of this program?

Mindful Eating (Chapter 8): This skill involves applying observing, adopting a nonjudgmental stance, and focusing on one thing in the moment to eating. It means slowing down, focusing on each bite of food with full awareness, consciousness, and attention to each moment, each taste, each chew. It is the opposite of binge eating in that when you eat mindfully you are in touch with your values and are committed to your long-term best interests.

❑ Are you taking advantage of the skill of mindful eating to help stop a binge from progressing or to stop urges to binge?

Urge Surfing (Chapter 8): This skill uses mental imagery to visualize your urge to binge as if it were a wave on the ocean. You use the mindfulness skills of observing, focusing on one thing in the moment, and adopting a nonjudgmental stance to "surf" this wave, or "surf" your urges to binge eat by staying with the experience of the urge without succumbing to it or intensifying it (by judging it or yourself).

❑ Are you practicing urge surfing to detach yourself from your urges, so that your brain learns it is possible to experience an urge without acting on it?

Mindfulness of Your Current Emotion (Chapter 9): This skill involves being fully aware of and open to the current moment, accepting all of your emotional experience and rejecting none of it. Using the mindfulness skills of observing, focusing on one thing in the moment, and adopting a nonjudgmental stance, you can externalize and remain separate from your emotion while still maintaining an awareness of it.

❑ Are you practicing mindfulness of your current emotion as a way to cope with strong emotions? This includes not attempting to suppress, block, or push your emotion away, and also not attempting to intensify it.

Radically Accepting Your Current Emotions (Chapter 9): This skill will help you tolerate emotions that you find difficult and thus give you options other than binge eating. The word *radical* is Latin for "root," and *radically* accepting your emotions involves accepting your feelings at their root or core in a deep and fundamental way. By accepting your emotions instead of fighting them, you can turn your attention to determining what you may be able to change about the situation that is causing the emotion and at the same time accept what you cannot change.

❑ Are you remembering to practice this skill as an alternative to binge eating when you encounter difficult situations and emotions that you find hard to accept?

Decreasing Vulnerability/Building Mastery (Chapter 10): The acronym PLEASE is intended to help you remember to treat P*hysica*L *illness,* balance your E*ating,* A*void* mood-altering substances, balance your S*leep,* and get E*xercise.* Building mastery involves doing activities that increase your sense of competence and confidence.

❑ Are you remembering to identify ways to reduce the vulnerabilities that ultimately lead to binge eating?

Building Positive Experiences (Avoiding Avoiding) (Chapter 11): Many individuals who binge eat have an imbalance in their lives, experiencing more unpleasant or neutral events than pleasant or satisfying events. This skill recognizes the importance of prioritizing positive experiences as a way to decrease your vulnerability to your emotion mind and to binge eating.

Are you practicing this skill by doing the following:

❑ Increasing the frequency of pleasant activities every day?

❑ Working on your long-term goals?

❑ Attending to your current relationships, setting boundaries in relationships that feel harmful to you, and reaching out to build new relationships?

❑ "Avoiding avoiding" by actively blocking your use of avoidance and binge eating to escape dealing with life's problems?

(continued)

Being Mindful of Positive Emotions (Chapter 11): This skill involves focusing (and refocusing) your attention on positive experiences when they occur and not becoming distracted through secondary reactions like worry, guilt, or self-criticism that can undercut your pleasant experience.

❑ Are you remembering to practice this skill so that you experience the pleasant events in your life as fully as possible, thus reducing your vulnerability to distressing emotions and urges to binge?

Half-Smiling (Chapter 12): This skill aims to facilitate an inner acceptance of reality through changing your external facial expression. Fully relaxed facial muscles, with a slight upturn of your lips (a serene, not tense, slight smile), changes the feedback to your brain.

❑ Are you taking advantage of this powerful skill by half-smiling during situations in which you lack control, at least in the moment (e.g., being stuck in traffic, waiting on a long line), increasing your acceptance and thus reducing your urges to binge?

Crisis Survival Skills (Chapter 12): These skills are intended to help you tolerate painful events and emotions when your other skills have "gone out the window." They are not designed to solve the problem. Instead, they help you get temporary relief to make it through the crisis or emergency without making matters worse.

To help you through a big or small crisis without turning to food, are you practicing the following crisis survival skills:

❑ Distracting (e.g., by shoring yourself up during an intense situation with an activity like exercise or a hot shower) so that you'll be able to respond effectively when there is an opportunity to do so?

❑ Self-soothing, or using the five senses to nurture or soothe yourself?

❑ Thinking of pros and cons, or thinking, in a very deliberate way, about the advantages and disadvantages of tolerating your distress versus the advantages and disadvantages of binge eating?

Coping Ahead (Chapter 13): This skill involves mentally rehearsing, as specifically as possible, how you would use your skills to cope with an upcoming difficult situation. Using this skill helps increase the likelihood that, when you actually face the situation, you will know how to respond skillfully.

❑ Are you practicing this powerful skill, rehearsing in detail what you will actually say and what you will actually do, so that you'll be less likely to turn to binge eating?

EXERCISE 2 Skills You Plan to Use More Often

Read through the list of skills taught in this program on pages 241–244. Are there any **skills** that stand out as ones you think might be **useful for you to use more often?** If a more in-depth description of the skill might be helpful, turn to the chapter in which it is discussed.

In the space that follows, list the top three skills that you would like to use more often.

1. _____

2. _____

3. _____

Kat wrote:

1. *Half-Smiling*

2. *Urge Surfing*

3. *Focusing on One Thing in the Moment*

Evaluating Your Progress

EXERCISE 3 Plotting Binge Episodes since Completing Chapter 7

a. **Collect your completed Diary Cards so that you can review your progress in stopping binge eating from the halfway point (Chapter 7). Count up and list below the number (if any) of binge episodes you had each week,** beginning at the point at which you completed Chapter 7.

To be consistent with how you counted these episodes in Exercise 2 of Chapter 7, count either the total number of large binges each week or the total number of large plus small binges. If there were days when you did not fill out your Diary Card, just use your best guess.

We're assuming, as we did in Chapter 7, that you're reading approximately one chapter every week, which would currently place you at about Week 13 of the program. If that isn't the case, write in the week that you're actually at. For example, Kat (see her progress evaluation on the next page) began her evaluation at Week 10 and is now on Week 17.

Week 8 _____   Week _____

Week 9 _____   Week _____

Week 10 _____   Week _____

Week 11 _____   Week _____

Week 12 _____   Week _____

Week 13 _____   Week _____

Week _____   Week _____

Kat wrote:

Week 10 __*0*__   Week *17* __*0*__

Week 11 __*0*__   Week _____

Week 12 __*1*__   Week _____

Week 13 __*0*__   Week _____

Week *14* __*0*__   Week _____

Week *15* __*0*__   Week _____

Week *16* __*0*__   Week _____

b. **Plot the number of binge episodes on the vertical axis** on the graph below, just as you did in Chapter 7's Exercise 2.

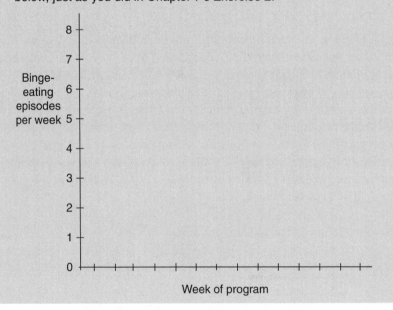

Kat drew:

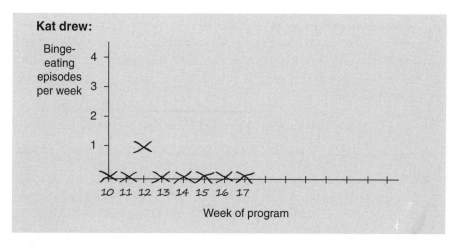

EXERCISE 4 Describing Your Binge Eating Trend over Time

Now, looking at either the graph or just at the numbers you have written down, describe any trends you observe. Has there been a decrease? An increase? A choppy pattern of increases and decreases? Or have the numbers stayed pretty much the same?

_____

_____

Kat wrote:

_Ever since the halfway point in Chapter 7, when I realized I was not put-
ting the same effort into this program that I had when I started, and my
binge eating validated that observation, I have felt more motivated. I also
changed things so that I had more time to read and do the exercises and
homework. Since then, my binge eating has decreased again, eventually
stopped, and stayed stopped. I also have really gotten a lot out of the new
skills I've learned in this second half of the program._

EXERCISE 5 What Have You Learned about Your Binge Eating
and Your Typical Triggers, Vulnerabilities, and Links
since the Halfway Point?

Review the Behavioral Chain Analysis Forms you have filled out since beginning Chapter 8.

a. **Typical prompting events** (e.g., dinner party, argument). List **the most common prompting events you've experienced** since beginning Chapter 8. If you completed Exercise 5 in Chapter 7, have your typical prompting events changed, or are you still struggling with the same ones? Record your answer below.

_____

_____

_____

_____

_____

_____

_____

_____

_____

_____

_____

_____

Kat wrote:

My main trigger is still one of the ones that I wrote about in Chapter 7—having leftovers after hosting a dinner party. But it rarely turns into a binge these days. The one time it did, which was during Week 10, was when I didn't get enough sleep the night before. I actually gave away almost all the leftovers to my guests, but I still had a small binge on the leftovers I had planned to save as a treat for the next day. I didn't ask my husband to help me clean up after the party because he was tired too and we hadn't been getting along that well. I also didn't practice urge surfing or mindful eating. In retrospect, I would have done better if I had not cleaned up that evening and had just gone to bed. I think I was just too vulnerable.

One of my previous main triggers from Chapter 7, looking in the mirror, no longer leads to binge eating. I feel good that I've been able to use the skills of adopting a nonjudgmental stance and radically accepting my emotions to cope a lot more effectively with the shame I feel when I look in the mirror. It's a lot less intense now.

Interestingly, my husband's withdrawal from me is also no longer a *trigger, because we are communicating much more often and directly. But the consequence of having more frequent and direct communication is that we are fighting a lot more.*

b. **Typical vulnerability factors** (e.g., overtired, alcohol, stress). List your typical vulnerability factors. Have the plans you made in Chapter 10 to address them been effective? If not, what are your plans to modify them?

_____

_____

_____

_____

_____

_____

_____

_____

_____

_____

Kat wrote:

Like I was mentioning, I have really learned that not getting enough sleep makes me far more vulnerable to my emotion mind. For the most part, though, I have been following through on my plans to get more sleep—and also to drink less caffeine. So while they are still vulnerability factors, they don't come up as frequently. But when they do, they are still a problem. As I write this, I'm remembering that on the night of the party I drank too much coffee as I was preparing the food because I could tell I was tired. I am particularly vulnerable on days when I have a lot to do, like hosting a party. My plan for that is to be more aware and keep using the worksheet on decreasing vulnerabilities. I think my vulnerabilities sneak past me and it's only in retrospect that I can identify them. If I were more aware ahead of time, I would be more able to access appropriate skills to deal with the situation or remove myself from situations that are too tempting.

c. **Typical dysfunctional links** (e.g., feeling anxious and thinking "I can't stand this without eating," feeling anger with the thought "I deserve this," feeling overwhelmed with the thought "I know the skills are there but I just don't want to use them," and/or feeling demoralized with the thought "What the heck? Why even try?"). What are your **typical dysfunctional links?** How do they compare with those you've had at earlier points in the program? Describe below.

_____

_____

_____

_____

_____

_____

_____

_____

_____

Kat wrote:

In the past my typical dysfunctional links had to do with feelings of intense shame about myself. But now they are more about anger that comes up when I am not being treated fairly, particularly by my husband. We are communicating more, as I said, but also fighting more. This is making me more anxious about whether or not our marriage can survive. But I feel good that I am not binge eating in response to this. I am trying to stay present and authentic.

Planning for the Future

Coping Ahead to Prevent a Binge

The last skill we're going to teach is coping ahead, a powerful tool that involves rehearsing a plan ahead of time for emotionally intense situations before they come up—so that you are prepared to cope skillfully. A key to making coping ahead effective is using visualization in a particular way that's borrowed from sports psychology. For mental rehearsal to be effective to improve basketball free throws, for example, the athlete has to visualize the basketball in his hands, visualize the basketball hoop, and then visualize the ball leaving his hands and sinking into the hoop. If the athlete takes on the perspective of a bystander in the stands or someone filming from above and watches himself as he throws the basketball, the mental rehearsal does not have the same positive effect on actual athletic performance. Therefore, as you mentally rehearse coping ahead, visualize yourself inhabiting your body as you practice skills, not visualizing as if you were watching a movie of yourself practicing skills. Coping ahead requires that you literally go through the motions.

Coping ahead can be used when you want to rehearse ahead of time for situations that, in the past, triggered you to binge—such as those you described in Exercise 5. With coping ahead, you face the same difficult situation you did in the past but this time visualize yourself turning to the skills instead of to food. Practicing the skill of coping ahead increases the likelihood that you will respond more automatically and skillfully, thus preventing yourself from binge eating when actually facing the situation for which you have practiced. Indeed, mental rehearsal can be as effective as actually physically practicing a skill.

A point we want to emphasize is that our approach in this program has been to teach you to become your own DBT coach. The program includes skills, like the behavioral chain analysis, that help you think more effectively about your binge-eating behaviors. Instead of feeling demoralized and giving up if you have had a binge, we hope you have learned to adopt a nonjudgmental stance and have experienced the empowerment that comes from identifying patterns that led to past difficulties. Understanding what made you vulnerable and what emotions triggered you gives you the opportunity to substitute skillful behaviors, such as coping ahead, so that you no longer remain stuck repeating past patterns.

EXERCISE 6 Practicing Coping Ahead

Step 1: To practice coping ahead, think of a future situation in which you will be at increased risk of binge eating. It might be an actual upcoming event (e.g., a party to which you have been invited) or simply a situation you are likely to face (based on past experience) that it would benefit you to be ready for, such as one of the prompting events you listed earlier in Exercise 5.

Situation (describe):

_____

_____

_____

_____

_____

_____

Kat wrote:

I am thinking about a difficult situation being a dinner party in the future like the one I experienced recently. Both my husband and I are tired and maybe not getting along all that well, so I don't feel comfortable asking for his help to clean up afterward. Though I wrote before that in those instances I should just go to sleep, that is not completely realistic. There will be some food I will have to clean up so we don't get ants and our pets don't get into it. Being around all of the leftover food, even if I am able to wrap up most of it and have my guests take it with them, will be incredibly tempting.

Step 2: Identify the emotion(s) that you will be experiencing and any urges to binge eat or turn to any other problem behavior. Be as specific as possible.

_____

_____

_____

_____

_____

_____

_____

_____

_____

Kat wrote:

I will be feeling resentful at my husband if he is relaxing and getting ready for bed while I am cleaning up. I may even start to worry he doesn't love me enough to want to help—that I'm not worth it, not deserving or valuable enough. Experiencing a mixture of resentment and shame, I will likely experience strong urges to binge. On top of these emotions, I might also experience the letdown I often feel after we host a party. I end up missing the excitement of having the house filled with people and conversation and don't know how to calm myself down after everyone has gone. I will likely feel physically uncomfortable, kind of amped up, even though I will be tired. I will have an urge to eat the leftovers, knowing that eating will calm me down, at least temporarily, and distract me from my resentment and anxiety about my husband and my loneliness and letdown about cleaning up after the party by myself.

Step 3: Visualize using coping ahead to practice a skill or skills that you think would help prepare you to cope with this emotion or an associated urge. See yourself in detail practicing turning to the skills. As you do, observe to see if any obstacles come up. If so, cope ahead with those obstacles. Describe your practice of this skill below.

_____

_____

_____

_____

_____

_____

_____

_____

_____

_____

_____

_____

_____

_____

_____

_____

_____

_____

_____

_____

Kat wrote:

This was interesting to do. I can see it would be useful, but it was hard to stick with it. My attention wandered at times, and I had to keep bringing myself back to what I was doing. Also sometimes I found myself watching myself. It helped to picture this like a video game where there is a choice to take on the perspective of the avatar—seeing everything through her eyes (but she can't see herself)—or to view the entire scene, like an aerial view. I kept wanting to watch the party like it was a movie instead of practicing this skill, rehearsing being myself in the future.

I started out looking at my guests, waving good-bye to them as they left. Right away I practiced diaphragmatic breathing to slow myself down. As I was breathing, I then practiced being effective. I found myself focusing on my goal, which was to clean up without binge eating. I kept breathing and then practiced adopting a nonjudgmental stance. By not judging myself or my situation, I actually noticed myself feeling more willing to consider alternatives to my earlier assumption that my husband found me unlovable or didn't want to help me. In this visualization, I found myself trying to remember if maybe I even told him I would just clean up everything myself.

If I keep practicing using coping ahead with these skills, I think I would not get to the place where I feel so worthless that my emotion mind tells me there is nothing to do but binge. That would break the chain.

Just to be prepared, though, I practiced coping ahead for the possible situation of being in the kitchen, putting away the leftovers, and experiencing an urge to binge even though I had practiced diaphragmatic breathing and being effective earlier. I visualized using the crisis survival skill of distracting with intense sensations and putting a hot washcloth over my face in the bathroom near the kitchen. This gave me time to access my wise mind. I practiced being effective and going to my husband to let him know I'd really appreciate his help cleaning up.

For the amped-up feeling, I visualized using a self-soothing skill and making myself a cup of tea. I checked to see if I still felt any urges to binge in order to calm down. If I sensed them, I visualized going to the coping ahead plan with the washcloth with hot water so I could calm down enough to focus on being effective and asking my husband to help me.

Angela's Practice of Coping Ahead

Angela told us that she had noticed a pattern of binge eating when she returned from traveling with her husband and children after vacations. To help break this pattern, she practiced coping ahead with Exercise 6. For Step 1, the situation she chose was returning from a planned 1-week vacation that was 3 weeks in the future.

For Step 2, she identified her emotions as feeling irritable, grouchy, and resentful about how much of the work (e.g., unpacking the suitcases, starting the laundry, tending to the pets, making a meal, beginning to prepare things for the next day of work and school) always seemed to fall on her shoulders. In addition to identifying her emotions, she identified typical vulnerability factors—feeling tired, jet-lagged, and almost always feeling hurt and disappointed about an interaction or two with a family member over the vacation that hadn't gone well. In terms of her urges, she typically experienced urges to binge on leftover candy that her family purchased at the airport for the trip, but that her children hadn't finished.

For Step 3, Angela used coping ahead to vividly visualize landing at the airport with her family, driving home, and then unloading suitcases from the car into their home. She visualized practicing half-smiling and noticed, as she did, that she felt more open to and accepting of the reality of the end of vacations being a difficult time. She also visualized using her diaphragmatic breathing. Both of these skills helped her feel calmer, and her urges to eat the candy decreased. However, as she continued to put away clothes and do other chores, she visualized herself feeling resentful and experiencing increased urges to "treat" herself with the candy. She visualized practicing urge surfing, which was one of her favorite skills, until the urge decreased. She then visualized continuing to do chores and noticing that the resentment returned, as had the urge to binge on the candy. She practiced seeking guidance from her wise mind. In her visualization, her wise mind advised her to think dialectically. Angela practiced accepting her desire to put her feet up and binge on all the candy and to accept how important her commitment to stop binge eating and feel good about herself in the morning were to her. This felt helpful. She visualized consulting her wise mind again and being advised to take a break and eat a meal with her family while practicing mindful eating. Angela then practiced decreasing her vulnerability to her emotion mind by taking a nap so she didn't get overly tired. She also visualized practicing building positive experiences by scheduling a pleasant activity with her husband after she awoke, watching a television show they both enjoyed. Angela breathed deeply as she fully imagined giving herself permission to enjoy this pleasant event, fully focusing her attention on her pleasurable emotions and refocusing on them if she becomes distracted by guilt or worry. She felt calm, took several more breaths, and ended the coping ahead exercise.

You can use coping ahead not only when anticipating situations with which you've had difficulty in the past, but also to imagine new situations where you're not sure which skills might work best. Coping ahead allows you to imagine the upcoming circumstances, including different scenarios in which you try different skills. So that you'll be as prepared as possible, you might visualize practicing one skill and then, if it doesn't work, visualize yourself trying another. You might find it useful to practice visualizing yourself in a situation in which your urges are so strong that you don't want to use any skills—and then visualize what might help in that same context (e.g., having your 3" × 5" card accessible to remind you of your top reasons for stopping binge eating, or a voice recording you made about how much binge eating has interfered with your values, pulling out a pros and cons worksheet, looking at a list of your top crisis survival skills). As we mentioned, coping ahead or mentally visualizing yourself practicing the skills makes it more likely that when you are in the actual situation, you will automatically follow through.

If You Start Binge Eating Again (or if Your Binge Eating Worsens Significantly)

We now want you to use the skill of coping ahead to plan how you would prevent yourself from relapsing if you started to binge eat again (or, if you haven't completely stopped at this point, if your binge eating were to worsen significantly). This may sound like an odd thing to "plan" for. But remember the skill of dialectical thinking. You can simultaneously be completely committed to not binge eat while also having a plan for what to do if you did binge.

First, though, we want to make clear that there is a big difference between a lapse (or slip)—a temporary return to binge eating—and a relapse—a full-blown return to binge eating.

A simple example of a coping ahead plan if you had a lapse into binge eating is to visualize that you'd use the skills of observing, adopting a nonjudgmental stance, and being effective to write out a behavioral chain analysis of the episode. This would enable you to understand what led to the binge and would provide a structure for creating a plan to prevent yourself from feeling so stuck and demoralized that the lapse would turn into a relapse. The behavioral chain analysis would include identifying skills you could use so that, when faced with similar triggers and links, you could act differently and break the chain leading to the binge. You could also use the behavioral chain analysis to identify and address your vulnerability factors. Your plan might also include rereading the book (or a particular chapter, such as Chapter 2 or 7), and/or beginning to fill out Diary Cards and Behavioral Chain Analysis Forms on a regular basis.

Exercise 7 asks you to come up with your own coping ahead plan. If you think it would be helpful, you may wish to look at the examples of coping ahead plans from Leticia and John (see pages 257–258) as guides before writing yours.

EXERCISE 7 Plan for Coping Ahead If You Start Binge Eating Again (or If Your Binge Eating Worsens Significantly)

How would you cope effectively with a future binge (or worsening of other problem behaviors) so that you do not feel stuck and move from a lapse into a relapse? Use coping ahead to describe the specific skills you would use (Hint:

don't forget to adopt a nonjudgmental stance!) to help yourself get back on track and stay on track in the future. Write your plan below.

_____

_____

_____

_____

_____

_____

_____

_____

_____

_____

_____

_____

_____

Leticia's Plan for Coping Ahead If Her Binge Eating Returns

Well, it has happened. I had the best of intentions, but things have slipped a little and I'm having binges again. First things first. I need to remind myself that critical judgments are not going to help me. Making myself feel bad about bingeing has never helped in the past and it certainly won't help this time. I also need to remember that all the skills I learned to stop binge eating haven't disappeared. I still have them; they may have merely collected a little dust from disuse. I just need to put together a plan to start reading the program again (a chapter a week), just to review everything. Right away, though, I need to start doing behavioral chain analyses for the binges I've had and generate ways to interrupt them using all the skills that I have learned. I need to remember, too, that a lapse is not the same as a relapse.

When I first worked through this program, I found dialectical thinking, urge surfing, and mindfulness of my emotions to be extremely helpful. I would want to start using these skills in particular while I work through the program again. Also, I almost forgot, the commitment!!! It was very helpful to write the commitment down on a card and put it in my purse, carrying it with me wherever I went. I will get that going right away. And remember, be kind to yourself, Leticia. It is the judgments that often turn one binge into many. So, be kind to yourself, learn from this binge, and keep moving forward!

John's Coping Ahead Plan If He Starts to Binge

If I start having difficulty with my eating, I will need to make time to check whether I've stopped using my skills or whether I need a refresher because I've stopped using some that I really need to start using again.

1. I visualize myself making copies of the Diary Card and putting them next to my bed so that I'm reminded to fill them out every day. Then I picture myself filling them out every day till I start to feel like I'm back in control.

2. I visualize myself looking at the DBT emotion regulation model from Chapter 1. In the big picture, I ask myself, what emotions am I finding hard to manage without turning to food? I'm guessing one might be shame, triggered by being critical/judgmental with myself. The skills I'm going to use will be radical acceptance and adopting a nonjudgmental stance. I remind myself that my goal is to be aware of these feelings. I don't have to make them go away. I can just notice them without having to change them. That helps me, as does thinking about how I would treat others. I would be much less critical and would validate their right to feel the way they do.

3. Another uncomfortable emotion for me to tolerate is my desire, how much I want something. It's hard for me to deprive myself, especially of food when I feel that I deserve it as a reward, like after a long day at work and then a business dinner. I will use the skills of mindful eating, and I can also decrease my vulnerability by balancing my eating so that I'm eating at mealtimes instead of skipping lunch, as I tend to do when I get busy. I also can practice mindfulness of my current emotion to help me as I'm observing my emotion as something separate from myself, like a river, while I sit on the bank. That has been helpful in allowing me to tolerate my feelings, including desire, without having such strong urges to turn to food as a way to cope with them. I can also look over the other skills I know from this program.

4. Last, I need to think about the big picture of my life and what I want and deserve. Feeling self-respect is more satisfying than the temporary satisfaction of excess food. When I was making time for this program, I felt

Barriers to Continuing to Live the Life You Want

Often, we find that as people have started using the skills in this program, their overall quality of life has improved. Sometimes, though, they uncover other issues that need to be dealt with. This section asks you to think about potential barriers to continuing to build the life you want to live.

EXERCISE 8 Barriers to Continuing to Live the Life You Want

List any barriers to **continue building a satisfying and rewarding quality of life for yourself** below.

_____

_____

_____

_____

_____

_____

_____

_____

_____

_____

_____

_____

_____

_____

Kat wrote:

Since I have stopped binge eating and am feeling as if I have greater self-esteem, I have noticed that I am feeling a great deal of anger toward my husband. Although I am feeling better about myself and my appearance, my anger is interfering with my ability to feel close to him. I have been socializing more, and developing relationships with people who are feeding the artistic side of me, but I know that I still need to work on my marriage in order to really live the life I want. I am going to approach my husband and suggest couples therapy to see if we can deal with some of these issues.

Question: Now that the program is over, do I need to continue to complete a daily Diary Card and a Behavioral Chain Analysis Form each week?

Answer: The truth is that these decisions are completely up to you. What is most important is that you are regularly reminded to use your skills instead of turning to food. If filling out your Diary Card each day and/or completing behavioral chain analyses on a regular basis has been helpful so far, it makes sense to continue these practices.

Question: Should I continue practicing all of the skills? Or is it OK to just practice some of them? Should using the skills feel fully automatic by now, so that I don't really need to "practice" them anymore?

Answer: Whether you decide to continue practicing some or all of the skills is another choice that is up to you. The bottom line is that in our experience, people who stop using the skills have been more likely to find their old ways of seeing, experiencing, and being in the world come back, and often, binge eating is a result.

This program is really about teaching you a new way of being and responding in the world. We expect you will use the skills you have learned to help you continue to live in this new way. We hope you've seen that the skills become easier to turn to the more you make them a part of your life. However, it may remain an effort for you to use them rather than to turn to food. We hope you agree that, in the long run, putting in the effort to use the skills is well worth it.

Chapter 13 Summary

The overall purpose of this chapter was to offer you a chance to reflect on your progress throughout this program. We reviewed the rationale behind this program's approach and highlighted the importance of continuing to practice the skills. We then asked you to review the skills as well as the progress you have made with stopping binge eating. We also asked you to review the situations that make you vulnerable to binge eating and how you plan to address them. This included teaching you how to cope ahead, a skill to use whenever you fear you may be entering a situation that places you at risk of binge eating. Coping ahead gives you a way to mentally rehearse using skills so that you will be more likely to turn to them automatically when faced with the actual situation. The last section of this chapter focused on looking toward the future. We asked you to use coping ahead to make a plan to address your binge eating if it were to return or increase. We then asked you to identify any barriers to continuing to build a satisfying and rewarding quality of life for yourself.

Homework

Remember to check the box after you have completed each homework assignment.

HOMEWORK EXERCISE 13-A
Committing to the Future

We hope that you have learned the power of making a commitment and that you will now decide to make a new commitment—to not binge eat *and* to continue to use this program and your skills in the future.

Take a moment and decide whether or not you wish to make this commitment. If you are unsure, you may want to review the pros and cons of making the commitment and not making the commitment.

Use the space below to write down your commitment.

Commitment to Not Binge Eat *and* Turn to This Program in the Future

_____

_____

_____

_____

_____

❏ I have recommitted to not binge eat and to turn to this program in the future.

❏ I'll remember to listen to my wise mind and get the most out of my life!

Congratulations!

Congratulations on working through this program and on the commitment you made to stop binge eating and live a fuller life—one in which you feel more able to live up to your potential and experience the richness in yourself and in the world without the numbing and deadening effects of binge eating or other problem behaviors. We truly wish you to have the highest quality of life possible. With the commitment and dedication to a better future you've shown by completing this program, the world is full of possibilities for you.

APPENDIX

What Studies Form the Basis for This Program?

To date, five clinical trials investigating DBT adapted for treating eating disorders form the basis for this program. The first, by Telch and colleagues (2000) included women with binge-eating disorder who received DBT in weekly group therapy delivered by trained therapists. This small trial showed quite good results, with 82% of the 11 participants stopping binge eating by the end of the study and 70% maintaining those changes 6 months later. A second, larger study was performed in 2001. Forty-four women with binge-eating disorder randomly received group DBT or a wait-list control (Telch, Agras, & Linehan, 2001). A total of 89% receiving DBT stopped binge eating by the end of the study compared to 12% receiving the wait list. After 6 months, 56% of those who had received DBT continued to not binge eat.

In 2001, Safer, Telch, and Agras (2001) compared DBT delivered by a trained therapist in 20 individual sessions to a wait-list control for 31 women with bulimia nervosa. Those who received DBT significantly decreased their binges (27/month) and purges (40/month) from before treatment to the end of treatment (binges = 1.5/month; purges = 1.0/month). Individuals who received the wait list showed no significant decreases in binge eating or purging.

In 2010, a larger study involving 101 men and women with binge-eating disorder compared DBT delivered by a trained therapist in 20 sessions of weekly group therapy to a comparison therapy that focused on increasing self-esteem and self-efficacy (Safer, Robinson, & Jo, 2010). At the end of treatment, those in the DBT group were significantly more likely to have stopped binge eating (64% vs. 36%). Unfortunately, the 12-month findings were complicated by the fact that many more members of the control group had dropped from the follow-up assessments, with 24% missing data compared to only 2% in the DBT group. At 12 months after treatment ended, 64% of the DBT group continued to be free of binge eating compared to about 43% of the control group.

The preceding studies suggest that DBT adapted for binge eating and bulimia nervosa is an effective treatment when delivered by a trained therapist. The program outlined in this book was developed over the course of several years. To broaden the availability of DBT, we adapted the treatment manual used in the preceding studies. Instead of designing it for therapists to use with their patients (Safer, Telch, & Chen, 2009), we wrote it so that individuals like you could use it on your own or with the guidance of a therapist.

We tested this program (Masson, von Ranson, Wallace, & Safer, 2013) in a study involving 60 men and women with binge-eating disorder who were offered either guided self-help or a wait-list control. Guided self-help included receiving a manual, referred to as the Toolbox, which formed the basis for this book. Participants also had the option to receive up to six 20-minute phone conversations with a therapist who could answer any questions they had about how to use the manual. After 13 weeks, 50% of those who not only received but also finished the entire DBT guided self-help Toolbox had completely stopped binge eating (Masson, 2012). Of those who received the DBT guided self-help Toolbox and started but did not necessarily finish the entire program, 40% had completely stopped binge eating when measured after 13 weeks. In comparison, only 3% of those who were on the wait list for 13 weeks had completely stopped binge eating (Masson et al., 2013). Six months later, 75% of those who had stopped binge eating at 13 weeks with DBT remained binge free. Even patients who did not completely stop binge eating with DBT significantly decreased their binge eating, on average. Such promising results suggest this program is an effective treatment option for binge eating.

A recently funded study (Carter-Major, Heath, Adler, & Safer, 2016) enabled us to expand our previous guided self-help study. The new study compares outcomes for binge eaters who receive this DBT program as either guided self-help or pure (unguided) self-help to binge eaters who receive a non-DBT treatment (compassion-focused therapy for binge eating).

References

Carter-Major, J., Heath, O., Adler, S., & Safer, D. L. (2016). *A randomized controlled study of a dialectical behavior therapy guided self-help intervention for binge eating disorder*. Study funded by the Newfoundland and Labrador Centre for Applied Health Research.

Masson, P. C. (2012). *A randomized wait-list controlled trial of dialectical behaviour therapy guided self-help for recurrent binge eating: A pilot study*. Unpublished doctoral dissertation.

Masson, P. C., von Ranson, K. M., Wallace, L. M., & Safer, D. L. (2013). A randomized wait-list controlled pilot study of dialectical behaviour therapy guided self-help for binge eating disorder. *Behaviour Research and Therapy, 51*(11), 723–728.

Safer, D. L., Robinson, A. H., & Jo, B. (2010). Outcome from a randomized controlled trial of group therapy for binge eating disorder: Comparing dialectical behavior therapy adapted for binge eating to an active comparison group therapy. *Behavior Therapy, 41*, 106–120.

Safer, D. L., Telch, C. F., & Agras, W. (2001). Dialectical behavior therapy for bulimia nervosa. *American Journal of Psychiatry, 158,* 632–634.

Safer, D. L., Telch, C. F., & Chen, E. Y. (2009). *Dialectical behavior therapy for binge eating and bulimia.* New York: Guilford Press.

Telch, C. F., Agras, W. S., & Linehan, M. M. (2000). Group dialectical behavior therapy for binge-eating disorder: A preliminary, uncontrolled trial. *Behavior Therapy, 31,* 569–582.

Telch, C. F., Agras, W., & Linehan, M. M. (2001). Dialectical behavior therapy for binge eating disorder. *Journal of Consulting and Clinical Psychology, 69,* 1061–1065.

Resources

References

Agras, W. S., & Telch, C. F. (1998). The effects of caloric deprivation and negative affect on binge eating in obese binge-eating-disordered women. *Behavior Therapy, 29,* 491–503.

American Psychiatric Association. (2013). *Diagnostic and statistical manual of mental disorders* (5th ed.). Arlington, VA: Author.

American Psychiatric Association. (2013). *Guideline watch (August 2012): Practice guideline for the treatment of patients with eating disorders* (3rd ed.). Washington, DC: Author.

Fairburn, C. G. (2013). *Overcoming binge eating: The proven program to learn why you binge and how you can stop* (2nd ed.). New York: Guilford Press.

Kabat-Zinn, J. (2013). *Full catastrophe living: Using the wisdom of your body and mind to face stress, pain, and illness* (rev. ed.). New York: Bantam Books.

Linehan, M. M. (1993). *Cognitive-behavioral treatment of borderline personality disorder.* New York: Guilford Press.

Masson, P. C. (2012). *A randomized wait-list controlled trial of dialectical behaviour therapy guided self-help for recurrent binge eating: A pilot study.* Unpublished doctoral dissertation.

Masson, P. C., von Ranson, K. M., Wallace, L. M., & Safer, D. L. (2013). A randomized wait-list controlled pilot study of dialectical behaviour therapy guided self-help for binge eating disorder. *Behavior Research and Therapy, 51*(11), 723–728.

Miller, W. R., C'de Baca, J., Matthews, D. B., & Wilbourne, P. L. (2001). *Personal values card sort.* Albuquerque: University of New Mexico.

Safer, D. L., Robinson, A. H., & Jo, B. (2010). Outcome from a randomized controlled trial of group therapy for binge eating disorder: Comparing dialectical behavior therapy adapted for binge eating to an active comparison group therapy. *Behavior Therapy, 41,* 106–120.

Safer, D. L., Telch, C. F., & Agras, W. (2001). Dialectical behavior therapy for bulimia nervosa. *American Journal of Psychiatry, 158,* 632–634.

Safer, D. L., Telch, C. F., & Chen, E. Y. (2009). *Dialectical behavior therapy for binge eating and bulimia.* New York: Guilford Press.

Sysko, R., & Walsh, B. T. (2008). A critical evaluation of the efficacy of self-help interventions for the treatment of bulimia nervosa and binge-eating disorder. *International Journal of Eating Disorders, 41,* 97–112.

Telch, C. F., Agras, W. S., & Linehan, M. M. (2000). Group dialectical behavior therapy for binge-eating disorder: A preliminary, uncontrolled trial. *Behavior Therapy, 31,* 569–582.

Telch, C. F., Agras, W., & Linehan, M. M. (2001). Dialectical behavior therapy for binge eating disorder. *Journal of Consulting and Clinical Psychology, 69,* 1061–1065.

von Ranson, K. M., & Robinson, K. E. (2006). Who is providing what type of psychotherapy to eating disorder clients? A survey. *International Journal of Eating Disorders, 39,* 27–34.

Organizations Providing Information on Eating Disorders, Dialectical Behavior Therapy, Dietary Guidelines, and Healthy Eating

Eating Disorders

UNITED STATES

National Eating Disorders Association (NEDA)
200 West 41st Street, Suite 1203
New York, NY 10036
Telephone: 800-931-2237
Website: *www.nationaleatingdisorders.org*
E-mail: *info@NationalEatingDisorders.org*
   Offers information and referrals, literature, and eating disorders screening.

Binge Eating Disorder Association (BEDA)
637 Emerson Place
Severna Park, MD 21146
Telephone: 855-855-2332
Website: *http://bedaonline.com*
   Provides outreach, education, and advocacy to increase awareness, proper diagnosis, and treatment of binge-eating disorder.

Academy for Eating Disorders (AED)
11130 Sunrise Valley Drive, Suite 350
Reston, VA 20191
Telephone: 703-234-4079
Website: *www.aedweb.org*
E-mail: *info@aedweb.org*
   A global professional organization that provides education on eating disorder symptoms and treatment.

Eating Disorders Resource Center (EDRC)
15891 Los Gatos Almaden Road
Los Gatos, CA 95032
Telephone: 408-356-1212
Website: *http://edrcsv.org*
E-mail: *info@edrcsv.org*
   Provides resources to the public and health professionals for early detection, intervention, and treatment of eating disorders. Advocates for mental health parity and effective insurance coverage.

Anorexia Nervosa and Related Eating Disorders (ANRED)
Website: *www.anred.com*
E-mail: *jarinor@rio.com*
   An objective resource for information on anorexia nervosa, bulimia, binge-eating disorder, and other less well-known eating disorders.

CANADA

National Eating Disorder Information Centre (NEDIC)
200 Elizabeth Street, ES 7-421
Toronto, Ontario M5G 2C4, Canada
Telephone: 866-633-4220
Website: *http://nedic.ca*
E-mail: *http://nedic.ca/nedic-feedback*
   A nonprofit that provides resources on eating disorders and weight preoccupation.

Bulimia Anorexia Nervosa Association (BANA)
1500 Ouellette Avenue, Suite 100
Windsor, Ontario N8X 1K7, Canada
Telephone: 519-969-2112
Website: *www.bana.ca*
E-mail: *info@bana.ca*
A nonprofit charity and community-based organization that advocates for eating disorder awareness and treatment.

Eating Disorders Association of Canada/ Association des Troubles Alimentaires du Canada (EDAC-ATAC)
E-mail: *edacatac@gmail.com*
A Canadian organization of professionals in the field of eating disorders.

UNITED KINGDOM

National Health Service
Website: *www.nhs.uk/Conditions/Eating-disorders/Pages/Introduction.aspx*
The eating disorders web page on the official site of the National Health Service, offering comprehensive health information about eating disorders and health care services, including clinical research trials.

Royal College of Psychiatrists (RCPsych)
21 Prescot Street
London E1 8BB, United Kingdom
Telephone: 020 3701 2552
Website: *www.rcpsych.ac.uk/expertadvice/ problemsdisorders/anorexiaandbulimia. aspx*
This website offers information about anorexia nervosa and bulimia nervosa.

Men Get Eating Disorders Too (MGEDT)
c/o Community Base
113 Queens Road
Brighton, BN1 3XG, United Kingdom
Website: *http://mengetedstoo.co.uk*
E-mail: *sam@mengetedstoo.co.uk*
An organization that aims to provide information and advice about eating disorders that is specific to men's needs.

Beating Eating Disorders (B-eat)
(formerly the Eating Disorders Association)
Wensum House
Unit 1 Chalk Hill House, 19 Rosary Road
Norwich, Norfolk NR1 1SZ, United Kingdom
Telephone: (adults) 0808 801 0677; (youth under 25) 0808 801 0711
Website: *www.b-eat.co.uk*
An organization that supports anyone affected by eating disorders or issues with food, including families and friends.

IRELAND

The Eating Disorders Association of Ireland (Bodywhys)
P.O. Box 105
Blackrock, County Dublin, Ireland
Telephone: 1890 200 444
Website: *www.bodywhys.ie*
E-mail: *info@bodywhys.ie*
Offers support, awareness, and understanding for people with eating disorders in Ireland.

AUSTRALIA

Eating Disorders Victoria (EDV)
Collingwood Football Club Community Centre, Level 2
Lulie and Abbot Streets
Abbotsford, Victoria 3067, Australia
Telephone: 1300 550 236 or (03) 9417 6598
Website: *www.eatingdisorders.org.au*
E-mail: *edv@eatingdisorders.org.au*
A comprehensive source of information on eating disorders, including early warning signs, services, and information on supporting someone with an eating disorder.

National Eating Disorders Collaboration (NEDC)
Level 2, 103 Alexander Street
Crows Nest, NSW 2065, Australia
Telephone: 1800 33 4673
Website: *www.nedc.com.au*
E-mail: *info@nedc.com.au*
Provides information on the prevention and management of eating disorders in Australia.

Dialectical Behavior Therapy

Behavioral Tech, A Linehan Institute Training Company
1107 NE 45th Street, Suite 230
Seattle, WA 98105
Telephone: 206-675-8588
Website: *http://behavioraltech.org*
E-mail: *info@behavioraltech.org*
Offers resources on DBT for mental health professionals and the community, including referrals for local DBT providers, mindfulness resources, and other information.

British Isles DBT Training
Website: *www.dbt-training.co.uk*
Provides information on training in DBT within Great Britain and the Republic of Ireland.

Dialectical Behaviour Therapy.com
Website: *http://dialecticalbehaviourtherapy.com*
E-mail: *info@dialecticalbehaviourtherapy.com*
Offers information on DBT resources in Australia.

Websites Providing Dietary Guidelines

UNITED STATES

Choose My Plate
USDA Center for Nutrition Policy and Promotion
3101 Park Center Drive
Alexandria, VA 22302–1594
Website: *www.choosemyplate.gov*
Offers information on USDA dietary and nutrition guidelines.

UNITED KINGDOM

NHS Choices: Food and Diet
National Health Service
Website: *www.nhs.uk/Livewell/Goodfood/Pages/Goodfoodhome.aspx*
E-mail: *www.nhs.uk/aboutNHSChoices/Pages/ContactUs.aspx*
Provides information about food, diet, and healthy eating.

IRELAND

Healthy Eating Guidelines
Healthy Ireland
Website: *www.healthyireland.ie/health-initiatives/heg*
Provides information from Ireland's Department of Health on guidelines for healthy eating.

AUSTRALIA

Australian Dietary Guidelines
Website: *www.eatforhealth.gov.au*
E-mail: *dietaryguidelines@nhmrc.gov.au* or *health@nationalmailing.com.au*
Offers guidelines and publications on healthy eating.

Size Diversity and Healthy Eating

Health at Every Size (HAES) and Association for Size Diversity and Health (ASDH)
P.O. Box 3093
Redwood City, CA 94064
Telephone: 877-576-1102
Website: *www.haescommunity.org*; *www.sizediversityandhealth.org*
E-mail: *contact@sizediversityandhealth.org*
Organizations dedicated to the practice of health at every size, an evidence-based approach to health that shifts from a focus on weight control to health gains and advocates against weight discrimination.

Health at Every Size UK
Website: *https://healthateverysize.org.uk*
Information on Health at Every Size as a means of promoting well-being and fostering size acceptance through equality and compassionate self-care.

Health at Every Size Australia
Website: *http://haesaustralia.weebly.com*
Provides information, training, and specialist availability regarding Health at Every Size in Australia.

Index

Note. *f* following a page number indicates a figure.

About the Authors

Debra L. Safer, MD, is Associate Professor of Psychiatry and Behavioral Sciences at Stanford University School of Medicine and Codirector of the Stanford Adult Eating and Weight Disorders Clinic.

Sarah Adler, PsyD, is Clinical Assistant Professor of Psychiatry and Behavioral Sciences at Stanford University School of Medicine and a clinical psychologist in private practice.

Philip C. Masson, PhD, is on the Adjunct Clinical Psychology Faculty at Western University and is a psychologist practicing in London, Ontario, Canada.

Drs. Safer, Adler, and Masson have worked with over 1,000 adults and adolescents with eating and weight concerns, with a focus on DBT and other evidence-based treatments.